INSIDE OUT

The essential women's guide to pelvic support

Michelle Kenway
Dr Judith Goh

Michelle Kenway is a consulting physiotherapist at the Mater Private Hospital—Redlands Women's Health Unit. She is a highly qualified and experienced private practitioner, women's exercise instructor and educational presenter. **Dr Judith Goh** is a Urogynaecologist based at Greenslopes Private Hospital; and Professor, School of Medicine Griffith University, Queensland.

Inside Out
The essential women's guide to pelvic support

Copyright © Michelle Kenway 2009

First published 2009
Reprinted 2012

Published by Healthy Fit Solutions Pty Ltd

All rights reserved. No part of this book, stored in any retrieval system or transmitted in any form or by any means, electronic, mechanical, photocopying, recording or otherwise without prior permission in writing by the authors.

ISBN 978 0 646 50889 4

Photography Mark Lobo
Illustrations Karen Mounsey-Smith
Designed by Sunset Publishing Services Pty Ltd

The information in this book is intended as general information and is not a substitute for medical consultation or advice. Consult your doctor before beginning this or any other exercise program. Whilst the authors have undertaken to ensure the accuracy of the material in this book, no promise expressed or implied concerning the content is made. The authors accept no risk of liability for any loss any person may suffer directly or indirectly by having relied upon the information provided in this book. All names and personal accounts in this book are fictional.

Foreword

Exercising and staying relatively fit should be encouraged at any stage of our lives. We are all aware that exercise has numerous benefits including reducing the risk of various medical conditions. Pelvic floor dysfunction, including urinary incontinence and pelvic organ prolapse, is common and becomes increasingly common as women age. Pelvic floor dysfunction is not confined to the older woman, and many younger women are also affected.

Women with pelvic floor dysfunction often have a desire to exercise but find that certain exercises exacerbate their symptoms. In fact, some women actually present to the gynaecologist after joining the gymnasium because they find that they now leak urine with exercise or feel that there is a vaginal prolapse. Many of the exercises and gymnasium machines are designed for those without risk of pelvic floor problems. Women with or at risk of pelvic floor dysfunction should be encouraged to stay healthy and in a normal weight range. They should also be advised that due to pelvic floor weakness, exercises are not prohibited but should be encouraged.

There is a great need for the information contained in this book to assist women who want to exercise without a negative effect on the pelvic floor. Pelvic floor exercises are vital in maintaining a healthy supportive pelvic floor. This book is an excellent educational tool for women of all ages.

Professor Judith Goh
Greenslopes Private Hospital

Contents

Foreword   Judith Goh   iii

Introduction   Michelle Kenway   vii

SECTION I   GET YOUR INSIDES INTO GEAR   1

1   All about your insides   2
    Understand what holds you up and in control—your pelvic floor and abdominal muscles.

2   Tone up your pelvic floor   11
    Discover the secrets for getting your pelvic floor into peak condition.

3   Take control of your abdominals   22
    No more sit ups! Flatten the appearance of your stomach and improve your control.

4   Exercise and pelvic floor problems   27
    Common place pelvic floor problems and tips for pelvic floor safe exercise.

SECTION II   SHAPE UP YOUR BODYWORK   36

5   Improve your fitness and lose your fat   37
    Get fit with aerobic fitness exercise that is kind to your pelvic floor.

6   Get your body strong—active workouts   46
    Get strong, tone up and stay young with strength exercises to protect your pelvic floor.

7   Gym and equipment exercises exposed!   65
    Exercise with confidence by doing what you should and avoiding what you shouldn't.

8   Exercise classes and your insides   71
    What to choose and what to avoid—how to participate in and avoid the pelvic floor
    pitfalls of exercise classes.

9   Home, class or exercise centre?   80
    Confused about your options for your health and fitness? Tips to help you make the
    best choices for your pelvic floor and the long-term success of your exercise program.

References   87

Introduction

DO YOU NEED HELP TO REGAIN CONTROL OF YOUR BODY?

Let me introduce you to Linda, age 52 . . .

> By the time I finally got the courage to tell someone about it and seek help I felt like my body was falling apart and I was losing control. I was depressed about the way I looked and felt, and the fact that I could no longer exercise. I had stopped exercising six months earlier owing to my embarrassing leakage and then piled on an extra 7 kg, mostly around my middle. I felt like a failure . . .
>
> (Chapter 5)

Does this story sound familiar? Linda is typical of the many thousands of women over 40 who are confronted by physical challenges and are desperate to take back control over their own bodies. Many women suffer in silence owing to the effects of menopause, including decreased bladder control and vaginal prolapse. Pelvic floor issues can make you feel very vulnerable, depressed and as though you are aging fast.

Some women say they are just too frightened to exercise for fear of embarrassing symptoms or making their pelvic floor condition worse. Exercise is particularly important for women in preventing a range of diseases, increasing fitness and energy levels, decreasing body fat, managing stress and depression, and much more . . . You can exercise and you can address your health problems and be a more active woman who is in control, by knowing what to do and how to do it!

Many women who are exercising and trying to look after themselves are actually damaging their insides and making their symptoms much worse through the wrong kind of exercise. Until recently, it was assumed that strength and fitness exercises suitable for men were also suitable for women, and very often both sexes are still prescribed similar exercise programs today. We are now finally realizing that some popular exercises are just not suited to a mature woman's pelvic floor, which is vulnerable and susceptible to injury. We want you to know the secrets to exercising your body safely and really effectively, so that you can feel great about yourself, in total control of your body, and confident that you can avoid injury and embarrassing symptoms.

> *My first baby was a big boy (9 lb 5 oz). He was a forceps delivery. My body has never been the same since. I have always loved exercising, it makes me feel good. Recently I started to notice a bulging heavy feeling in my vagina especially after the gym and I was absolutely devastated when my GP told me that that I had a prolapse and that I had to stop heavy exercise. I cried all the way home. I was so humiliated. I had no idea that childbirth and the wrong kind of exercise could affect me this way.*
>
> Carol, age 47 (Chapter 7)

IS YOUR WHOLE BODY CHANGING? DO YOU NEED PROFESSIONAL EXERCISE GUIDANCE?

Life events such as childbirth and menopause are often accompanied by unexpected physical changes, especially over 40 years of age. Changing hormones associated with menopause can have a debilitating effect on your body. You may have noticed a loss of strength and tone, and that you become easily fatigued. Your body fat may have increased, especially around your waist. Maybe you notice that when you sneeze you leak a little. You may have been told by your doctor that you are at risk of a disease that can be addressed through appropriate exercise. Perhaps you are stuck in a rut of inactivity and weight gain, and although you want to exercise you just don't know how to safely go about it.

DO YOU HAVE PROBLEMS WITH YOUR PELVIC FLOOR WHEN YOU EXERCISE?

Maybe you leak or pass wind when you run or jump, making exercise embarrassing and unpleasant. You may find that when you are active you need to rush to the toilet frequently. Perhaps you have been diagnosed with a vaginal prolapse and that some types of exercise cause a bulging, heavy and uncomfortable feeling in your vagina. You may have already had a surgical repair for your pelvic floor problems. If this is you, then you are a woman who will benefit from professional exercise guidance!

ALL WOMEN ARE AT RISK, SOME MORE THAN OTHERS...

Unfortunately, our female anatomy places us all at risk of pelvic floor problems. Any of the following risk factors will further increase your risk of pelvic floor problems, particularly with the wrong kind of exercise: pregnancy, childbirth, constipation and straining, carrying too much weight, heavy lifting, chronic coughing, chronic lower back and/or pelvic pain, previous hernia repair, increasing age, and having a family history of incontinence and/or prolapse. If this sounds like you, then you are also someone who will benefit from the right professional exercise advice.

EMPOWERING YOU TO TAKE CONTROL OF YOUR HEALTH AND FITNESS

This book has been written to help you improve your pelvic support and exercise with confidence and control. The following chapters teach you how to take control over your long-term health through appropriate exercise for your body. You will read real life stories about how Linda and others like her overcame their health and fitness challenges through the right kind of exercise. You will learn about your unique physical female make-up. You will discover the secrets of pelvic floor and abdominal muscle exercises that really work to help you to improve your continence, support your insides and even flatten the appearance of your stomach. You will know how to be fit and lean with aerobic fitness exercise that is kind to your insides. You will be guided through a program of strengthening exercises that will improve your overall muscle strength, tone and energy as you protect your pelvic floor. You will be shown how to make the right exercise choices for your body so you can exercise with confidence, avoid injury, and achieve your own personal health and fitness goals.

Most of us are increasingly aware of just how essential exercise is for us to lead a long, active and healthy life. If you've been confused about how to exercise safely and successfully, now is the time to get active and make a start. Read on for your comprehensive guide to exercise for pelvic support.

Michelle Kenway

In memory of my wonderful mum

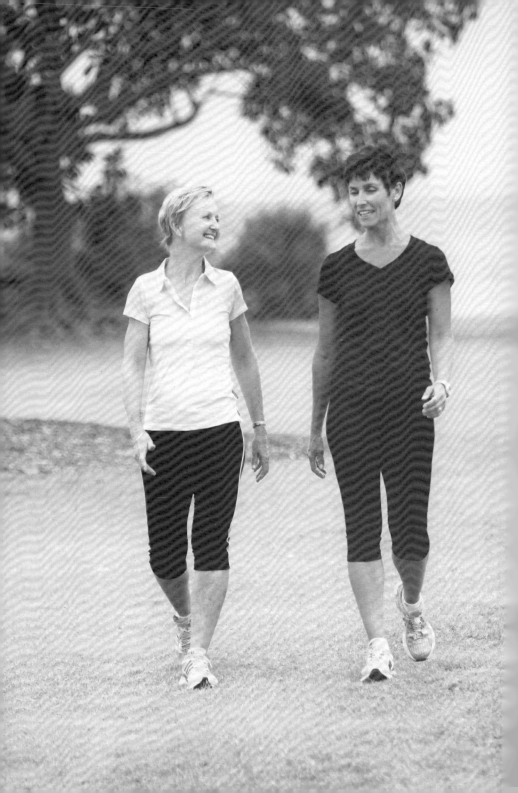

GET YOUR INSIDES INTO GEAR

1 All about your insides

YOUR PELVIC FLOOR

The pelvic floor is a mystery to many women, partly because it is located inside the body and hidden from view. Your pelvic floor spans the base of your pelvis in and around the area where you sit. It is made up of muscles, strong tissues, nerves, blood vessels, and the organs within your pelvis.

Your pelvic floor muscles are like a supportive hammock suspended between your pubic bone at the front and your tailbone at the back, as shown in Figure 1.1. These muscles sit in layers, covered and reinforced by strong tissues which attach to the inside walls of your pelvis. Different parts of your pelvic floor muscles encircle your urethra (urine tube), vagina and anus (the opening to your back passage). In order to perform their important roles in your body, your pelvic floor muscles need to work together for long periods of time and have the ability to contract strongly and quickly when you need them to.

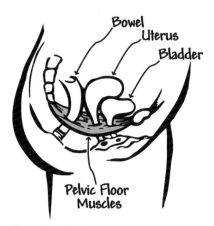

Figure 1.1 Pelvic floor muscles

WHAT DOES YOUR PELVIC FLOOR DO FOR YOU?

Holds your insides up and in

Your pelvic floor works to resist and counteract the constant pressure under which it is placed by everyday living. It supports your pelvic organs including your bladder, urethra, vagina, uterus and rectum (the final part of your bowel).

Keeps you dry and helps you to empty

It assists in storing and emptying wastes from your bladder and bowel.

Holds your body together

It works with other parts of your body to hold together or stabilize the bones of your pelvis and your spine.

Babies and the bedroom

It allows you to reproduce and contributes towards your sexual sensation and response.

WHAT CAN GO WRONG WITH YOUR PELVIC FLOOR?

Your pelvic floor is vulnerable to injury owing to its position in your body and the repeated pressure placed upon it on a daily basis. It can be affected by pregnancy and childbirth, changes with menopause and aging, specific health problems and lifestyle factors. Your inherited characteristics may also make you more susceptible to developing pelvic floor problems. Damage to your pelvic floor can result from a single episode of trauma to the area, or long-term events which repeatedly place downward pressure upon it. Repeated pressure onto a damaged pelvic floor can cause it to stretch and become floppy and weak. Alternatively, some women develop pelvic pain and pelvic floor muscle spasm which can also affect their ability to contract and relax these muscles. When your pelvic floor is not working well, it becomes less able to perform the important roles it plays, and your bladder, bowel and vagina may then lose their ability to function as they should.

Is your pelvic floor at risk?

If you answer yes to one or more of the following common risk factors, then you are a woman who is at increased risk of pelvic floor dysfunction.

☐ **I have had children ...**

During pregnancy and childbirth your pelvic floor muscles and tissues stretch and may become damaged, weak and lose sensation. Women who notice symptoms immediately following delivery may be more likely to experience problems later on. Sometimes, pelvic floor injuries related to childbirth do not become apparent until menopause and beyond.

☐ **I am going through/have gone through menopause ...**

Hormonal changes associated with menopause decrease the strength, endurance, thickness and elasticity of your pelvic floor tissues. These changes continue with increasing age after menopause.

☐ **I have a family history of pelvic floor problems ...**

Some of your inherited characteristics such as the elasticity and thickness of your tissues can increase your likelihood of pelvic floor dysfunction. Childhood bedwetting can also be a predictor of future problems with your bladder.

☐ **I never exercise my pelvic floor muscles ...**

When your pelvic floor muscles are not used they become thin and weak. Over time they may then become stretched and saggy, making it difficult for them to work together as they should.

☐ **I have experienced an associated health problem ...**

Chronic coughing, chronic lower back or pelvic pain, previous gynaecological surgery, pelvic radiation therapy, being overweight and long-term straining to empty your bowels all have the potential to affect the working ability of your pelvic floor.

☐ **I have an associated lifestyle factor ...**

The wrong kind of exercise, regular heavy lifting and the effects of smoking can also affect the ability of your pelvic floor to function as it should.

YOUR ABDOMINAL MUSCLES

Abdominal and pelvic floor muscles have been shown to work together in continent women.[1] If you do not use your abdominal muscles well or if you exercise them incorrectly, your pelvic floor can be affected.

HOW DO YOUR ABDOMINAL MUSCLES HELP YOU?

Work with your pelvic floor muscles

Your abdominal muscles should work appropriately with your pelvic floor muscles to support your pelvic organs and keep you dry.

Protect and support

Your abdominal muscles protect and support your abdominal organs.

Hold you together

Your innermost abdominal muscles wrap around your trunk and stabilize the joints in your spine and your pelvis. An added bonus is that when they work as they should, they may even flatten the appearance of your stomach!

WHAT CAN GO WRONG WITH YOUR ABDOMINAL MUSCLES?

Not enough ...

Your abdominal muscles can be used too little and stop working as they should. They can become stretched, injured, weak and inactive, making them unable to perform their important roles. This can be caused by factors such as pregnancy, being overweight, abdominal surgery, poor posture and chronic lower back pain.

Too much ...

If your abdominal muscles are used too strongly, they will create excessive downward pressure on your pelvic floor. Episodes of heavy lifting, straining, coughing, sneezing, vomiting, inappropriate abdominal exercises and pulling your tummy in too strongly can all force your pelvic floor downwards, **especially if it is weak**.

Just right . . .

If you can learn to use your abdominal muscles correctly, your pelvic floor will be able to better withstand the downward pressures associated with your everyday activities.

We are particularly interested in some specific abdominal muscles—those that are helpful and those that are not so helpful to your pelvic floor.

YOUR INNERMOST ABDOMINAL MUSCLES WORK WITH PELVIC FLOOR

Your abdominal muscles are positioned in layers. If you peel away the outer layers of abdominal muscles, you will find the deepest, innermost layer of your abdominal muscles called Transverse Abdominis. These deep muscles wrap around your trunk just like a corset. If you can imagine a corset covering your abdomen, wrapping around your waist and fastening at your spine, you will understand where these muscles lie. These deep muscles and their corset-like position are shown in Figure 1.2.

Your Transverse Abdominis muscles can be trained to work with your pelvic floor, to help support your insides and keep you dry. These muscles are designed to be gently active for long periods of time. It can initially take some time to find these muscles and use them correctly. You will learn how to take control of these muscles in Chapter 3.

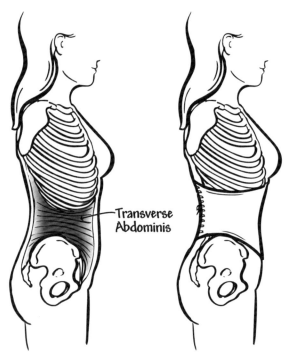

Figure 1.2 Deep abdominal muscles and corset-like arrangement

OUTER ABDOMINAL MUSCLES CAN HINDER YOUR PELVIC FLOOR

You are probably aware of at least one group of your outer abdominal muscles, your 'six pack' or Rectus Abdominis muscles. These strong muscles run vertically down your middle between your pubic bone and your rib cage. Your External Oblique muscles also make up your outermost layer of abdominal muscles. These outer abdominal muscles are illustrated in Figure 1.3.

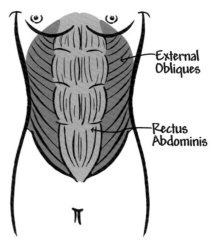

Figure 1.3 Outer abdominal muscles

Your outer abdominal muscles can have an adverse effect on your pelvic floor if you train or use them incorrectly. These muscles are designed to contract strongly, and they generate large amounts of pressure in your abdomen such as when you cough. If you think of squeezing a plastic sauce bottle, when you squeeze the sides of the bottle you increase the downward pressure inside the bottle and the sauce is forced out. In the same way, if you squeeze in your abdomen strongly, you increase the downward pressure upon your pelvic floor. If your pelvic floor is not strong enough to counteract this downward pressure, it will be forced downwards as shown in Figure 1.4.

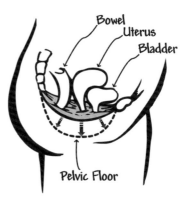

Figure 1.4 Pelvic floor forced downwards

This is the reason some women have symptoms when they use their outer abdominal muscles strongly, such as leakage when they cough. Interestingly, women who consciously try to flatten their stomach using these particular muscles can make their symptoms worse. These are definitely not the muscles to train to become stronger if you have or are at risk of pelvic floor problems. You may even need to learn NOT to use these muscles too strongly if that is what you are accustomed to doing.

Inside Out

YOUR CYLINDER OF SUPPORT

So far, you've learned that your pelvic floor and deep, innermost abdominal muscles should work together to help give you support and control your insides. The muscles surrounding your abdomen can be represented as the surfaces of a cylinder, as shown in Figure 1.5. The muscles making up your cylinder of support control the pressure in your abdomen.[2] Some of the muscles making up your cylinder of support include:

- ♀ your diaphragm (breathing muscle) which forms the lid of your cylinder
- ♀ your pelvic floor muscles which form the base of your cylinder
- ♀ your deep abdominal muscles which form the front of your cylinder and wrap around the sides to the back of your cylinder.

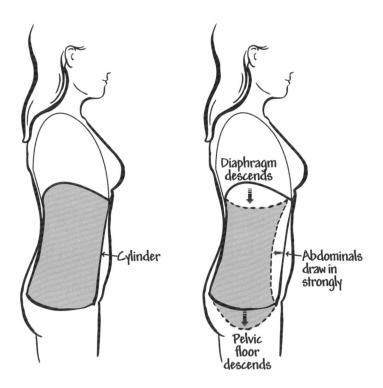

Figure 1.5 Cylinder of support (left) and the effect of excessive pressure causing your pelvic floor to descend (right)

All about your insides 9

If the muscles making up the lid, base or sides of your cylinder do not work together as they should, this can affect your ability to support your insides and stay dry. If your pelvic floor muscles do not contract when they should, pressure from within your abdomen can force your pelvic floor downwards as shown in Figure 1.5. This pressure can be caused by the front and sides of your cylinder squeezing inwards (i.e. your strong outer abdominals)[3] or the lid of your cylinder pressing downwards (i.e. your diaphragm). Your pelvic floor must be able to resist the pressure pushing down on it from above. If your pelvic floor cannot withstand this pressure, as a result of being forced downwards repeatedly over time it will become stretched and weak as shown in Figure 1.6. When this happens your pelvic floor becomes floppy and saggy, decreasing your ability to support and hold your insides in, close off your pelvic floor openings and stay dry.

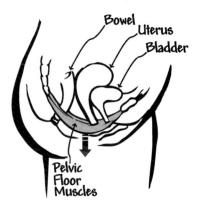

Figure 1.6 Stretched pelvic floor muscles

Key points about your insides

Your pelvic floor

- ♀ Is formed by muscles, strong tissues, nerves, blood vessels and pelvic organs
- ♀ Muscles span the base of your pelvis like a hammock
- ♀ Is involved in supporting your pelvic organs and resisting downward pressure, storing and emptying wastes, stabilizing your pelvis and spine, sexual reproduction and sexual response
- ♀ Can be affected by your age and stage of life, pregnancy and childbirth, disuse, inherited characteristics, specific health problems and lifestyle factors.

Your abdominal muscles

- ♀ Are positioned in layers
- ♀ Can lose their ability to work well and may be used incorrectly
- ♀ Deep, innermost abdominal muscles can assist your pelvic floor and should work together with your pelvic floor muscles
- ♀ Strong outer abdominals can create downward pressure and hinder your pelvic floor.

Your cylinder of support

- ♀ Your abdomen is surrounded by muscles in a cylinder-like arrangement.
- ♀ Your diaphragm, deep abdominal and pelvic floor muscles are some of the muscles forming your cylinder of support.
- ♀ Muscles making up your abdominal cylinder control the pressure in your abdomen and can affect your ability to close your openings and support your insides.
- ♀ Your pelvic floor must counteract the downward pressure from your abdomen; otherwise, if repeatedly forced downwards, over time it may become stretched, floppy and weak.

2 Tone up your pelvic floor

Many women find it difficult to contract their pelvic floor muscles when they first attempt pelvic floor muscle exercise. Perhaps you have never tried to use your pelvic floor muscles before, or you may not know how to even find these muscles, let alone exercise them. Adding to the challenge is the fact that you cannot see these muscles working from the outside of your body with the naked eye. It can be difficult to feel whether or not you are contracting your pelvic floor muscles if they are weak or if your sensation in this area is decreased. This chapter is designed to teach you how to find your pelvic floor muscles and, with the right kind of exercise, train them into their best possible condition.

It is never too late to start pelvic floor exercises. You can exercise and improve the condition of muscles that you can move voluntarily, regardless of your age. This includes your pelvic floor muscles. Pelvic floor muscle exercises will actually help you to counteract some of the changes to your pelvic floor associated with menopause and growing older.

HOW PELVIC FLOOR EXERCISE CAN IMPROVE YOUR CONTROL

As you have already read, your pelvic floor muscles can become stretched, floppy and weak. When this happens, things often start to go wrong, and sooner or later you will start to know about it. The right pelvic floor exercise can make your pelvic floor into a stronger, thicker and firmer support to hold up your insides, promote your ability to close off your pelvic openings, and control your bladder and bowel. Pelvic floor muscle training may also encourage your muscle hammock to sit higher inside your pelvis and improve your ability to actively incorporate these muscles into your every-day activities.

Training your pelvic floor muscles usually aims to improve your ability to:

- ♀ contract these muscles more strongly
- ♀ improve your ability to repetitively contract these muscles or to sustain a single contraction for longer; and/or
- ♀ use them in a timely and coordinated manner, such as contracting them briskly to counteract downward pressure before you sneeze.

IT WON'T HAPPEN OVERNIGHT . . .

The following pelvic floor muscle training program involves a number of stages. You should work through all three stages to get your pelvic floor into peak condition. Improvements in your pelvic floor fitness will commence even within the first couple of weeks of your exercise program, but it may take a little while longer before you start to notice the effects. To get your pelvic floor into its very best possible condition, you should commit to 5–6 months of dedicated exercise, particularly if your pelvic floor muscles are weak to start with. Try to stay focused on your goal of inner control, and remain committed and patient as your pelvic floor fitness improves.

STAGE 1: FINDING YOUR PELVIC FLOOR MUSCLES

My GP sent me to a physiotherapist to help me manage my prolapse. When my physio examined me and encouraged me to try to switch on my pelvic floor muscles I just couldn't do it. I had no idea what I was supposed to be doing and no matter how hard I tried, I just couldn't feel anything happening where I was supposed to be feeling it. It was really frustrating at first.

Carol, age 47

It can be extremely difficult to find your pelvic floor muscles and to know what a correct pelvic floor muscle contraction feels like. Unless you are certain about contracting your pelvic floor muscles correctly, you may perform the wrong exercise and make your symptoms worse. Stage 1 is essential to help you find your pelvic floor muscles and perform the correct action before you start practicing.

TECHNIQUES TO HELP YOU FIND YOUR PELVIC FLOOR MUSCLES

> A pelvic floor muscle contraction involves a squeeze of your pelvic openings (urethra, vagina and anus) and a lift up inside.

Choose from any of the following techniques to help you find your pelvic floor muscles:

Imagine

- ♀ Stopping the flow of urine once it has started and then restarting the flow
- ♀ Lifting up inside your vagina to resist withdrawing a tampon
- ♀ Stopping wind from passing by drawing up inside your anus
- ♀ Moving your tailbone forwards and up towards your pubic bone.

Look

- ♀ Lie on your side and use a mirror to look at the entrance of your vagina. You should see a tightening of the entrance of your vagina and a small inwards lift of your perineum (the area between your anus and vagina) as you contract your pelvic floor muscles.

Feel

- ♀ Sit on a rolled-up hand towel or the armrest of a lounge chair to feel the sensation as you squeeze your pelvic openings and lift up inside.
- ♀ Lie on your side with your knees bent, and use your index finger to touch your perineum and feel this area lift inwards away from your finger.
- ♀ Sit on an exercise ball and feel your pelvic floor muscles squeeze and lift up inside.
- ♀ Try gently drawing in your deep abdominal muscles as described in Chapter 3 and you may feel activity in your pelvic floor muscles at the same time.

TIPS TO HELP YOU ACTIVATE YOUR PELVIC FLOOR MUSCLES

You may initially find it easier to switch on your pelvic floor muscles:

- ♀ lying down either on your back, side, or kneeling forward while supporting your upper body through your elbows
- ♀ positioning your body with your knees close together before progressing to activating these muscles with your knees apart.

COMMON MISTAKES TO AVOID

Some mistakes are commonly made when women attempt to use their pelvic floor muscles. Try to avoid these common mistakes whilst contracting your pelvic floor muscles:

- ♀ Straining or pushing down instead of lifting inside
- ♀ Squeezing your buttocks and inside thigh muscles
- ♀ Drawing your outer abdominal muscles in strongly
- ♀ Holding your breath or changing your normal breathing pattern.

It is very important to have the correct technique before commencing practice. If you practice the wrong technique, you will potentially make your symptoms and condition worse. If you are still unsure or having difficulty activating your pelvic floor muscles after trying these suggestions, seek some professional guidance from a continence and women's health physiotherapist. A physiotherapist experienced in this field can provide you with the training, ongoing monitoring and motivation you may require to help you to rehabilitate your pelvic floor.

STAGE 2: TRAINING YOUR PELVIC FLOOR MUSCLES

Step 1 – Position

Start in the position you can best feel your pelvic floor muscles working. This may be lying down on your back, side or tummy if your muscles are not working well. Lying down helps to eliminate the effect of lifting against gravity and may make this exercise easier for you at first.

Step 2 – Posture

Always check your posture to ensure you have your lower back in its "neutral" position. This means that your lower back should be curved slightly inwards before and during your pelvic floor muscle contraction.

Step 3 – Squeeze, lift and breathe

Squeeze the muscles around your pelvic openings (your anus, vagina and urethra), and lift up inside. Continue breathing normally as you squeeze and lift. Do not hold your breath or change your regular breathing pattern—if you can't hold your pelvic floor muscles against a normal breath, you will never manage to hold them up against the much greater downward force of a cough or sneeze.

Step 4 – Relax

Slowly relax your pelvic floor muscles from their contracted position and return them back to their resting position. You should be able to relax your pelvic floor muscles after contracting them voluntarily.

Step 5 – Rest

Rest your muscles briefly before your next attempt.

YOUR PELVIC FLOOR MUSCLE TRAINING PROGRAM

Now that you can feel your pelvic floor muscles contracting with the correct action, you are ready to start training to get them into their best possible condition. You will need to *practice regularly* and *progress your exercises* to get your pelvic floor into top shape. The following clinical recommendations have been made regarding pelvic floor muscle training.[4]

1. Make each pelvic floor muscle contraction as **STRONG** as possible, maintaining your correct technique throughout.
2. Hold each strong contraction for 3–10 seconds.
3. Repeat 8–12 pelvic floor muscle contractions in a row (this is one full set).
4. Perform three sets of exercises each day.
5. Perform your pelvic floor muscle exercises **EVERY DAY**.

IF YOU CANNOT CONTRACT YOUR PELVIC FLOOR MUSCLES STRONGLY...

If your pelvic floor muscles are very weak, you may initially find it difficult to perform your exercises strongly and maintain the correct technique. It may be challenging to contract these muscles even for a couple of seconds. Do not despair, as pelvic floor training takes time, practice and patience! If your muscles are weak, commence with gentle contractions of your pelvic floor muscles and focus on using the correct technique. Start with the number of pelvic floor muscle contractions you can manage, and hold each contraction for as long as you can, even if only for one second at a time. Gradually try to increase how long you hold each contraction for, and the number of contractions you perform as you are able to. Try to make your muscle contractions stronger when you feel you can do so, but only when you can maintain the correct technique.

Tone up your pelvic floor

IF YOU ARE REALLY PRESSED FOR TIME ...

Some women report that they are just too busy to perform their pelvic floor muscle exercises daily. If you are one of these women, try to practice your exercises on at least three alternate days of the week. Ensure that you make each contraction as strong as possible to optimize the effectiveness of your exercises. Try to increase the amount of incidental exercise you can do, whether it be sitting waiting for an appointment or standing in a queue. Every bit of effective practice you do counts towards a healthier pelvic floor.

PROGRESSING YOUR EXERCISES

You will make your greatest improvements in strength during the first couple of months of training. It is very important that you progressively challenge your pelvic floor muscles to work harder to get your pelvic floor into peak condition. If you perform the same exercise program day after day, your strength and endurance will plateau instead of improving further.

Gradually progress your training to achieve your best possible pelvic floor fitness by:

- ♀ holding each contraction stronger
- ♀ holding each contraction for longer
- ♀ switching on your muscles faster
- ♀ loading your muscles with vaginal weights
- ♀ progressing the positions in which you exercise from lying down to upright.

Remember the key points for improving your pelvic floor fitness are:

1. Regular practice.
2. Progressively challenging your muscles to work harder.

STAGE 3: TRAINING YOUR PELVIC FLOOR MUSCLES FOR YOUR EVERYDAY ACTIVITIES

Congratulations, you are doing really well if you have been practicing and progressing your pelvic floor muscle exercises regularly! Now you need to start training your pelvic floor muscles to work in everyday activities, in both the positions and the situations you need them to work for you. If you do all your exercises lying down, your pelvic floor muscles will become trained to work for you in that lying-down position. This does not mean that they will work well for you standing up when you really need them to work.

Hi my name is Libby. At age 46 I was a fit and healthy person who exercised on a regular basis and enjoyed my life. Then I was diagnosed with cervical cancer and I was told I needed a Radical Hysterectomy. My whole life was turned upside down . . .

After my operation unfortunately the catheter needed to stay in for weeks. When it finally came out my pelvic floor was very weak and not functioning that well. When I coughed or lifted light weight, did anything, my bladder would leak. I started pelvic floor exercises that my physio gave me. I would practice any exercises that were possible when ever I had the opportunity like when I was standing in a queue at the supermarket, sitting at traffic lights, cleaning my teeth, standing and trying to listen to someone who I would rather not be listening to.

TRAINING IN DIFFERENT POSITIONS

As your pelvic floor fitness improves, your pelvic floor muscles become better able to work in upright positions. It is very important that you practice exercising your pelvic floor muscles in the positions that you need them to work. For most of us, this involves upright standing positions. Exercise your muscles in positions where you can feel your pelvic floor muscles working, and in the position that gives you a slight challenge to work a little harder.

Tone up your pelvic floor

A typical progression over a number of months may involve you training your pelvic floor muscles in the following increasingly challenging positions:

Lying down ➡ Sitting on a chair/towel roll/exercise ball with your knees together
⬇
Sitting with your knees apart
⬇
Standing with your knees close together
⬇
Standing with feet slightly apart or in stride stance
⬇
Semi-squat position with your hands resting on your knees as you lean forward slightly.

TRAINING YOUR MUSCLES FOR DIFFERENT ACTIVITIES

Try to practice using your pelvic floor muscles during specific activities every day, in addition to your prescribed exercise program. Many of your everyday activities place pressure on your pelvic floor without your even realizing it. You are more than likely to be aware of some of the activities that increase pressure on your pelvic floor, as these may cause symptoms such as leakage or vaginal heaviness. These are the types of activities that require you to incorporate pelvic floor muscle holds.

WHEN TO PRACTICE USING YOUR PELVIC FLOOR MUSCLES

You should practice using your pelvic floor muscles **immediately prior to and during** any activity that places pressure upon your pelvic floor. Unfortunately, the normal automatic activity of these muscles can be lost when your pelvic floor is damaged, which means they may not work when they are needed. You will benefit from activating your pelvic muscles before and during any activity that is potentially stressful for your pelvic floor. This will improve your ability to use these muscles when you really need them, as well as reducing your symptoms and protecting your pelvic floor from further injury.

Try to practice using your pelvic floor muscles with the following potentially stressful actions, particularly those that cause your pelvic floor symptoms. Practice using your pelvic floor muscles prior to and as you:

- laugh
- cough
- sneeze
- stand up
- bend forward
- step down.

MAINTAINING YOUR PELVIC FLOOR MUSCLE STRENGTH

Practicing your pelvic floor muscle exercises should be a life-long commitment. If you cease your exercises completely, you will lose the muscle improvements that you've worked so hard to achieve. When you know that you have trained to the very best of your ability and given yourself sufficient time to get your pelvic floor into the best possible condition, try to perform your exercises on at least one to two alternate days per week using the training program described. This will help you to maintain a healthy pelvic floor.

Key points for toning up your pelvic floor

- Pelvic floor muscle training can improve bladder control.
- Pelvic floor muscle rehabilitation takes at least 5–6 months for weak muscles.
- Pelvic floor muscles can be trained regardless of age.
- Avoid making common mistakes when activating your pelvic floor muscles.

Stages of pelvic floor muscle rehabilitation:

1. Finding your pelvic floor muscles

- ♀ Imagine, look and/or feel your pelvic floor muscles contract.
- ♀ A pelvic floor muscle contraction feels like a squeeze of your pelvic openings and an inwards lift.
- ♀ Attention to your position and posture will improve your muscle contraction.
- ♀ Seek professional guidance if you cannot find your pelvic floor muscles or perform the correct technique.

2. Training your pelvic floor muscle strength and endurance

- ♀ Practice using the correct technique.
- ♀ Commit to regular daily practice.
- ♀ Hold each contraction for 3–10 seconds.
- ♀ Each contraction should be as STRONG as possible.
- ♀ Practice 8–12 repetitions (1 set).
- ♀ Perform three sets per day (3 × 8–12 contractions).
- ♀ Commence with gentle contractions if your muscles are weak.
- ♀ Practice regularly, and progressively challenge your pelvic floor muscles to work harder.

3. Training your pelvic floor muscles for your everyday activities

- ♀ Practice using your muscles in different everyday positions.
- ♀ Practice using your pelvic floor muscles immediately prior to and during activities and actions that place pressure on your pelvic floor.
- ♀ Practice your exercises on at least one to two alternate days of the week to maintain a healthy pelvic floor.

3 Take control of your abdominals

Women often ask about the best exercises to flatten their stomach and narrow their waist. Weight gain in these areas is often associated with particular events in a woman's life such as pregnancy and menopause. Hormonal changes associated with menopause can actually cause a weight shift from the hips to the abdomen so that some women feel as though they suddenly develop a spare tyre around their middle. The great news is that if you can improve the control of your innermost deep abdominal muscles, you may assist your pelvic floor as well as flatten the appearance of your stomach. This chapter teaches you how to use your deep abdominal muscles well.

Before my bladder surgery I had been going to the gym for a couple of years. I had really wanted a flatter stomach. It didn't make any difference how many sit-ups I did, my stomach never changed. When I look back I think that this is about the time my leakage started getting worse.

Karen, age 49

No more sit-ups!

Stop the sit-ups! Sit-ups strengthen your outer abdominal muscles. Sit-ups are not helpful for your pelvic floor, and no matter how many you do they will never make your stomach flat. It is a common myth that sit-ups will flatten your stomach. It is not possible to spot-reduce fat with exercise. In fact, exercising your outer abdominal muscles may actually do you more harm than good. Doing regular sit-ups will repeatedly increase downward pressure on your pelvic floor. Strengthening your outer abdominal muscles may actually make them even more effective at increasing pressure upon your pelvic floor. This is how the wrong kind of abdominal exercise can worsen your pelvic floor symptoms and increase the likelihood of damage, especially if your pelvic floor muscles are already weak.

Take control of your abdominals

The correct abdominal muscles for most women to exercise are the corset-like deep abdominal muscles shown in Figure 1.2. These muscles can become stretched, weak and poorly used as a result of excess weight, pregnancy, lower back pain and poor posture. If you can use your deep abdominal and pelvic floor muscles together well, they can help you to reduce pelvic floor symptoms. Once again, these particular muscles are not visible from the outside of your body; however, you will see a gentle inward movement of your lower abdomen and a slight narrowing of your waist when you use them correctly. Exercising these muscles takes very little effort once you know how.

EXERCISING YOUR DEEP ABDOMINAL MUSCLES

Your deep abdominal muscles are postural muscles that are designed to work gently for extended periods of time. This means that this is the way you should train these muscles to work—gently and for long periods of time.

Step 1 – Posture

The first thing to do when learning to use your deep abdominal muscles is to attend to your posture. If your posture is slumped, you will not be able to use these muscles well. Either stand or sit in front of a mirror with your back away from the backrest of the chair. Lengthen your spine and lift your chest so that your body is tall, maintaining the small inward curve in your lower back as shown in Figure 3.1.

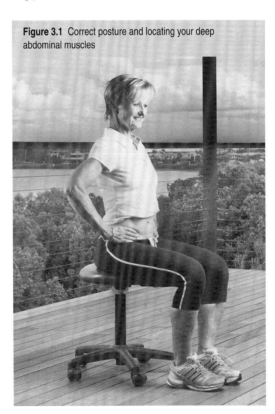

Figure 3.1 Correct posture and locating your deep abdominal muscles

Step 2 – Locate

Find your deep abdominal muscles by placing your second and third fingers inside your pelvic bones as if you were placing your fingers just inside both your hip pockets as shown in Figure 3.1. Keep your fingers positioned here as you activate these muscles.

Step 3 – Breathe

Breathe into the base of your rib cage (just above your waist level). As you breathe you should not see your shoulders and upper chest lifting. You should see the base of your rib cage widen and your abdomen move outwards as you breathe in. Breathe before and as you activate your deep abdominal muscles.

Step 4 – Activate

Contract your deep abdominal muscles by gently drawing in your lower abdomen towards your spine. This is the area of your belly beneath where your underwear sits. Your fingers should detect a slight tension and inward movement of your lower abdominal wall. When you activate these muscles correctly, you will see your waist narrow a little and your lower abdomen will flatten slightly. You may also feel some muscle activity develop in your pelvic floor muscles as you correctly activate these muscles. It is very desirable that you can feel both these groups of muscles working together.

Abdominal tip — Remember this is a very **gentle action**. DO NOT PULL YOUR STOMACH IN STRONGLY.

If you draw your belly in strongly, you will increase the downward pressure on your pelvic floor. If you can see your outer abdominal muscles tensing at the same time, you are pulling in your abdomen too strongly, as shown in Figure 3.2.

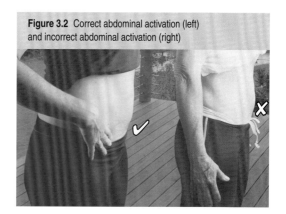

Figure 3.2 Correct abdominal activation (left) and incorrect abdominal activation (right)

Step 4 – Maintain

Initially, aim to keep these muscles contracted for 10–15 seconds at a time, for a minimum of 10 times per day.

Step 5 – Relax

Relax your deep abdominal muscles when you feel you can no longer maintain your gentle muscle contraction. Rest briefly and try to repeat this exercise again.

PROGRESS YOUR DEEP ABDOMINAL MUSCLE TRAINING . . .

Hold for longer

Practice contracting your deep abdominal muscles for increasingly longer periods of time when you are able to. There is no limit to the length of time you can practice holding them for.

HOLD AND MOVE

When you can control these muscles in standing, try slowly walking with them gently contracted. If they relax or become fatigued, stop, rest briefly and then start again. Placing your hands over your lower abdomen as you walk may help you to feel whether these muscles are still active when you are learning to use them.

PRACTICE WITH YOUR PELVIC FLOOR MUSCLES

Ideally your pelvic floor and deep abdominal muscles should work together. Everyday you have numerous opportunities to practice using these muscles together. Activate and keep your pelvic floor muscles contracted as you gently tense your deep abdominal muscles.

Practice using your pelvic floor and deep abdominal muscles together when you:

- ♀ sit with your back away from the backrest of your chair, e.g. during morning tea, or while waiting for appointments, typing or watching TV
- ♀ stand, e.g. in a shopping queue or while washing up
- ♀ lift and carry, e.g. shopping, laundry, babies, small children, or luggage
- ♀ push or pull, e.g. a trolley, vacuum cleaner, mower or golf buggy.

Key points for taking control of your abdominal muscles

- Life events can cause your waist to thicken and your stomach to expand.
- Your abdominal muscles can become stretched, weak and poorly used.
- Your outer abdominal muscles are exercised with sit-ups, and these muscles can increase downward pressure upon your pelvic floor.
- Your deep abdominal muscles should work with your pelvic floor muscles.

Exercising your deep abdominal corset muscles

- Good posture is essential.
- Practice in upright positions when your back is not supported.
- Find these muscles inside your pelvic bones as if placing your fingers in your hip pockets.
- Practice gently drawing in your lower abdomen and maintaining this muscle contraction.
- You may feel some activity in your pelvic floor muscles as you contract these muscles; this is desirable.
- Breathe normally when using these muscles.
- Try to increase the length of time you can keep these muscles active.
- Practice using these muscles when you move.
- Initially aim to contract these muscles for 10–15 seconds at least 10 times per day.
- Practice using your deep abdominal muscles with your pelvic floor muscles during your everyday activities.

4 Exercise and pelvic floor problems

It is highly desirable for women to exercise throughout life. The tremendous benefits of exercise for general health and well being over the course of a woman's life mean that it should be encouraged from a young age. It is also extremely important to ensure your good pelvic health by exercising appropriately throughout your life as your body changes over time.

HOW EXERCISE CAN CAUSE PELVIC FLOOR PROBLEMS

There are times during the natural course of a woman's life when her pelvic floor becomes more vulnerable to injury and long-term dysfunction. Childbirth, the onset of menopause and with the natural course of aging the pelvic floor becomes more susceptible to injury through inappropriate exercise. These events often trigger a woman's realisation that she needs to exercise for her health and wellbeing. It is commonplace for the menopausal women with a little more time available to her, to launch into a new exercise program. Following childbirth new mums are often keen to regain their pre-pregnancy fitness and so commence a new exercise program. Many such programs concentrate on intense abdominal core exercises.

THE PROBLEM OF OVERLOADING THE PELVIC FLOOR...

Long-term pelvic floor dysfunction can result from inappropriate exercises when the pelvic floor is more vulnerable. When the pelvic floor tissues weaken, they lose their ability to support the pelvic organs (including the bladder, uterus and rectum). The increased pressure associated with some kinds of exercise that overload the pelvic floor can force it downwards as illustrated in Figure 1.4. The more intense this exercise is, the greater the downward force on the pelvic floor. When repeated over time and even with a single episode of particularly intense pressure, long-term pelvic floor injury and dysfunction can result.

THE PROBLEM OF OVER-BRACING THE PELVIC FLOOR MUSCLES ...

Pelvic floor problems can also occur when the pelvic floor muscles become overactive and develop increased muscle tension. Some intense core exercises can cause the pelvic floor muscles to contract and become unable to relax. This can also occur when a woman habitually braces her pelvic floor muscles. The pelvic floor problems that can result from increased pelvic floor tension include chronic pelvic pain, pain during sexual intercourse along with bladder and bowel problems.

WOMEN WITH NORMAL FUNCTION ARE ALSO AT RISK ...

Even women with a normally functioning pelvic floor are at risk with inappropriate exercises. Some women commence an exercise class or gym routine with normally functioning pelvic floor muscles. Over time the demands of intense core abdominal exercises or inappropriate strength training regimes can repeatedly stretch and strain her pelvic floor muscles increasing the likelihood of pelvic floor problems such as pelvic organ prolapse and incontinence. Alternatively high level core exercises can prevent her pelvic floor muscles from relaxing as they should. These overactive pelvic floor muscles then become shortened and tight, and much more susceptible to injury.

Section II of this book outlines in detail those exercises that are most likely to cause overloading and over-bracing of the pelvic floor muscles. Let's now look at some commonplace pelvic floor problems and tips for exercising with these problems.

EXERCISE AND SPECIFIC PELVIC FLOOR PROBLEMS

GENERAL EXERCISE PRINCIPLES

- ♀ Ensure that your pelvic floor muscles have the capacity to withstand the exercise you choose.

- ♀ Exercise should not aggravate your pelvic floor symptoms either during the course of exercise or following your session.

- ♀ Avoid those exercises with potential to overload your pelvic floor, particularly if your pelvic floor muscle function is lacking. These are typically high impact aerobic exercises, inappropriate strength exercises and techniques, and intense core abdominal exercises.

- ♀ Avoid or modify exercises that involve over-bracing of your abdominal and pelvic floor muscles. These are typically intense core abdominal exercises. Pelvic floor and abdominal muscles need to be trained to contract and relax back to their resting position.
- ♀ Choose pelvic floor safe exercises and techniques in order to protect your pelvic floor as you exercise.
- ♀ Attend to weight management through appropriate exercise and diet. Excess body weight has the potential to make the following specific pelvic floor problems worse.
- ♀ Prioritise your pelvic floor muscle fitness to promote good pelvic support and control for your chosen exercises.

PROLAPSE AND EXERCISE

When diagnosed with a prolapse, many women become fearful of exercise and confused about appropriate exercise selection. Understanding how to maintain fitness and manage body weight are often primary issues of concern. Weight management through appropriate exercise is vital when living with a prolapse since the more weight you carry, the more load and pressure you place upon your pelvic floor, and your prolapse.

The general exercise principles outlined in Section II apply to a range of prolapse conditions including: anterior vaginal wall prolapse (also known as bladder prolapse or cystocoele), uterine prolapse, vaginal prolapse, posterior vaginal wall prolapse (rectocoele), rectal and anal prolapse conditions.

TIPS FOR EXERCISING WITH A PROLAPSE:

- ♀ Perform low impact weight bearing exercises such as walking when your body (and your pelvic floor muscles) are not fatigued.
- ♀ A couple of daily 10–15 minute daily exercise sessions are just as effective for your fitness and can be more comfortable than one long exercise session.
- ♀ Manage your body weight well and try to avoid unnecessary weight gain to avoid unnecessary loading of your pelvic floor.
- ♀ If your prolapse is large try to participate in non weight bearing fitness exercises such as appropriate water-based exercise.

- ♀ Consider wearing quality support briefs while exercising to promote improved pelvic support.

- ♀ Discuss your suitability for using a pessary for exercise with your gynaecologist. A pessary is a device designed to support prolapsed tissue within the vagina. Many women find that their exercise-related prolapse symptoms are markedly decreased when exercising using a pessary for prolapse support. Some pessaries are designed to remain within the vagina for extended periods of time. Others are designed so that they can be inserted and removed as required for exercise and activity.

- ♀ Using a pessary device will not weaken your pelvic floor muscles. A pessary may even assist your pelvic floor exercise or kegel exercises by lifting your prolapse thereby allowing you to better elevate your pelvic floor muscles when exercising them.

INCONTINENCE AND EXERCISE

Women living with bladder and or bowel incontinence issues can find exercising very challenging and embarrassing. Unfortunately some women choose to avoid exercise all together thereby missing out on the health benefits associated with exercise.

Specific problems such as bladder or bowel leakage and/or urgency during exercise can be minimised through appropriate exercise selection. A combined approach of pelvic floor fitness exercise and astute exercise selection can often allow a woman to exercise despite these issues. Some women find that as their general strength and fitness improve with appropriate exercise, their incontinence problems lessen. Once again weight reduction is an important factor if you are overweight and living with these issues.

TIPS FOR EXERCISING WITH INCONTINENCE

- ♀ Proper hydration is important during and after exercise. Do not withhold fluid during exercise. Your body is constantly producing urine and fluid you drink during exercise takes time to process. Water consumed during exercise will rehydrate your body rather than make you leak urine.

- ♀ Try to perform general exercise when your pelvic floor is not fatigued. The pelvic floor is often fatigued by the end of the day and may not function as well for support and control.

- ♀ Time your exercise routine to coincide with the times you are least urgent. Some women find their urgency is worst at a particular time of the day. In this case aim to exercise when your urgency is most settled.

- ♀ Try to avoid consuming your known bladder or bowel irritants such as caffeine immediately prior to exercise.

- ♀ Avoid high impact exercise which can increase urgency and instead select appropriate low impact exercises.

- ♀ You may notice that your incontinence is worse at particular times of your monthly cycle (often during the week prior to menstruation). Anticipate these cyclical changes so that you are not caught off guard at these times.

- ♀ Consider trialling a continence device for exercise. Continence devices such as Contiform are readily available and can be used for bladder support during exercise and activity.

- ♀ If you wear protective continence products, choose quality continence pads or liners rather than sanitary pads which tend to be less absorbent.

GYNAECOLOGICAL SURGERY AND EXERCISE

Previous gynaecological surgery presents an exercise challenge for women who are usually at increased risk of future pelvic floor problems owing to their surgery. Pelvic organ prolapse surgery increases the likelihood of repeat prolapse. There is evidence to suggest that hysterectomy surgery may also increase the likelihood of future pelvic organ prolapse. Some women undergo incontinence surgery only to find that their leakage recurs upon recommencing general exercise.

> To ensure the long term success of your gynaecological surgery and to minimise the risk of additional problems arising, you need to understand how to perform pelvic floor safe exercises long-term.

TIPS FOR EXERCISING AFTER GYNAECOLOGICAL SURGERY

- ♀ Never recommence general exercise without your specialist's approval to do so.

- ♀ Full healing following gynaecological surgery takes three months on average for most women. Avoid recommencing your previous intense exercise program immediately following your six week check up. Your internal tissues will still be healing and your risk of pelvic floor injury increased at this time.

- ♀ Exercise during the first six weeks post-operatively aims to prevent or minimise decline in your physical condition and reduce the risk of post-operative complications. This is definitely not the time to undertake a new fitness program.

- ♀ Exercise in the immediate post-operative six week period is usually limited to a progressive walking program that should be provided by your treating doctor or physiotherapist.

- ♀ When recommencing general exercise make sure that you have read and understand the pelvic floor safe exercise principles for fitness, strength and exercise class participation described in detail in Section II.

- ♀ Your specialist should advise you when it is appropriate for you to recommence general exercise. This will vary according to various factors including your: surgical procedure, overall recovery, fitness level prior to surgery and the capacity of your pelvic floor to withstand the pressure associated with your chosen exercise.

- ♀ If you are unsure about how well your pelvic floor is functioning to support your internal organs, seek a women's health physiotherapy assessment before recommencing your exercise program. If your pelvic floor muscles are not functioning well and you resume exercises involving intense loading of your pelvic floor, then you run the risk of injuring your newly healed pelvic tissues.

- ♀ Many women now seek women's health physiotherapy treatment prior to their surgery with the goal of rehabilitating their pelvic floor to optimise their long-term pelvic floor support.

PELVIC PAIN AND EXERCISE

Pelvic pain associated with increased pelvic floor muscle tension is increasingly common but often poorly understood and undiagnosed. Gynaecologists and physiotherapists are treating increasing numbers of women with overactive pelvic floor muscles resulting from inappropriate exercise, particularly intense core exercises.

Unfortunately Western society's culture of abdominal exercise, along with the current emphasis on core strength exercises has contributed to the rise in the number of women developing overactive pelvic floor muscles and associated pelvic pain/pelvic floor dysfunction. Some popular exercise classes such as Pilates and gym-based exercises involve extremely high level abdominal and pelvic floor bracing. If you've ever experienced tight neck muscles you will know how painful and debilitating overactive muscles can be. This is just the same for the pelvic floor muscles when they are trained to contract strongly and never given the opportunity or taught how to relax. A pattern of overactive pelvic floor muscle activity becomes learned and a cycle of chronic pelvic pain can develop.

> Pelvic floor muscles should be trained to contract appropriately when required to counteract increased abdominal pressure and then to fully relax to an appropriate resting level. The pelvic floor and abdominal muscles should not be constantly braced.

TIPS FOR EXERCISING WITH PELVIC PAIN

- ♀ If you suffer from pelvic pain seek treatment from a physiotherapist trained in women's health. Your treatment will usually involve learning to relax your affected pelvic floor muscles.

- ♀ Cease pelvic floor or kegel exercises until you are advised to recommence them by your treating health practitioner. If you continue with pelvic exercises when you do not know how to relax your pelvic floor muscles, your pelvic floor muscle tension and associated discomfort will be likely to worsen.

- ♀ Cease intense core abdominal exercises, high impact exercises and intense strength training until you are advised to recommence these exercises by your treating health practitioner.

- ♀ Appropriate general exercise is usually an important aspect of comprehensively managing pelvic pain. It can assist with stress relief and minimise physical deconditioning during the course of treatment in women with pelvic pain.

- ♀ Low impact exercise such as water-based walking can be a useful starting point for women suffering from pelvic pain.

- ♀ Break up your daily exercise into short sessions rather than one long session. This may involve a short walk in the morning and another in the afternoon when you feel capable of doing this.

- ♀ Take the time to rest your body and relax your pelvic floor immediately following exercise. Pelvic floor muscle relaxation can often be enhanced by lying down, placing a pillow under your knees, using warmth over your lower abdomen and/or pelvic region and relaxed diaphragmatic breathing.

FUNCTIONAL PELVIC FLOOR FITNESS

Well functioning pelvic floor muscles will promote your ability to keep participating in general exercise with comfort and confidence. Your pelvic floor muscles need to be strong enough to withstand the exercises you choose. They need to be well-timed so that they can contract and protect your pelvic floor before and during more intense and demanding exercises. Pelvic floor muscles require endurance so that they can withstand repetitive and prolonged exercises. They also need to be able to relax back to their normal resting level following exercise, especially following intense or repeated core abdominal exercises.

The better your pelvic floor muscles function, the greater your ability to perform a wide variety of general exercises throughout your life and protect your pelvic floor. The stronger and fitter your body is, then the less pressure that will be placed on your on your pelvic floor in your everyday activities and during exercise. As your body changes over time, you may find that you are no longer able to take for granted the fitness of your pelvic floor. This is why women need to incorporate pelvic floor exercise as an essential component of whole body exercise programs.

Key points for exercise and pelvic floor problems

♀ Exercise for women is highly desirable and we want to encourage women to participate in appropriate exercise for their health and wellbeing.

♀ Inappropriate exercise presents two major risks for women with pelvic floor problems:
   1. Overloading of the pelvic floor
   2. Over-bracing of the pelvic floor muscles

♀ Some women with normal pelvic floor function develop pelvic floor problems from inappropriate exercise.

♀ Some commonplace pelvic floor problems place a woman at increased risk of pelvic floor dysfunction and can prevent them from exercising effectively:
   - Pelvic organ prolapse
   - Incontinence
   - Gynaecological surgery for prolapse, incontinence and/or hysterectomy
   - Pelvic pain with overactive pelvic floor muscles

♀ Functional pelvic floor fitness is a priority for all women to ensure their ongoing ability to perform general strength and fitness exercise.

SHAPE UP YOUR BODYWORK

5 Improve your fitness and lose your fat

Do you want to improve your fitness, lose weight and energize your body? It can be really frustrating and even depressing if exercise makes symptoms such as leaking and discomfort worse. Knowing how to promote good health through exercise whilst preserving your pelvic floor can be a tricky business. Get set to learn how to improve your whole body fitness whilst protecting your pelvic floor and minimizing your symptoms.

> *By the time I finally got the courage to tell someone about it and seek help I felt like my body was falling apart and I was losing control. I was depressed about the way I looked and felt, and the fact that I could no longer exercise. I had stopped exercising six months earlier owing to my embarrassing leakage and then piled on an extra 7kg, mostly around my middle. I felt like a failure. I was even leaking when I tried to walk. I had also stopped drinking anything before going out. My back pain was also becoming worse and I was waking up during the night and needing to get up to go to the toilet. I felt tired all of the time.*
>
> Linda, age 52

AEROBIC EXERCISE FOR YOUR BODY AND YOUR MIND

Aerobic exercise can conjure up sometimes alarming images of tights, leotards and unbearably loud music. Fear not, as this is not what you need to do to get fit. Aerobic exercise actually refers to any form of continuous exercise that increases the workload of your heart and lungs, and noticeably increases your heart rate. This is the type of exercise that will improve your stamina and your cardiovascular fitness. You should do aerobic exercise in addition to your general everyday activities.

The right aerobic exercise will actually help you overcome some of the changes to your body brought about by menopause. Aerobic exercise can:

- ♀ decrease your risk of serious diseases including heart disease, stroke, diabetes and some types of cancer
- ♀ improve your ability to control your weight and decrease your body fat (very important for decreasing pressure on your pelvic floor)
- ♀ increase your energy levels and your endurance
- ♀ decrease joint and muscle stiffness and pain
- ♀ improve your ability to think clearly
- ♀ reduce anxiety, depression and stress
- ♀ make you feel really good about yourself!

THE BEST AEROBIC EXERCISES FOR YOUR PELVIC FLOOR

Low-impact types of aerobic exercise are the best exercises to minimize stress on your pelvic floor. Low impact means that you keep at least one of your feet in contact with the ground at all times and avoid large, jarring forces through your legs. Choosing this type of exercise will allow you to develop your fitness (while minimizing symptoms such as leakage) and exercise effectively without worsening your condition.

You can select the types of exercise you enjoy from the following list of suitable low-impact exercises:

- ♀ Walking
- ♀ Swimming
- ♀ Cycling
- ♀ Water walking
- ♀ Aqua aerobics
- ♀ Bushwalking
- ♀ Dancing
- ♀ Low-impact exercise classes (these are discussed in detail in Chapter 8).

Improve your fitness and lose your fat

General tips for reducing the impact of aerobic exercise on your pelvic floor:

- ♀ Choose flat surfaces.
- ♀ Wear cushioned shoes.
- ♀ Avoid continuous exercise on hard surfaces.
- ♀ Exercise in the morning when you are not fatigued.
- ♀ Exercise in short bouts as opposed to a long session.

BE KIND TO YOUR BODY AND AVOID HIGH-IMPACT AEROBIC EXERCISE

Activities that involve both your feet being off the ground at the same time or stepping heavily are high impact. As your body changes with menopause and increasing age, it becomes less suited to withstanding high-impact activities. High-impact exercise will place stress on your pelvic floor (and your joints). This type of exercise may worsen your symptoms and can potentially stretch and strain your pelvic floor, especially with repeated impact over time.

Some examples of high-impact activities are:

- ♀ Running/jogging
- ♀ Jumping
- ♀ Skipping
- ♀ Volleyball
- ♀ Netball
- ♀ Basketball
- ♀ Stepping down (platform)
- ♀ Tennis (competition)
- ♀ Squash (competition)
- ♀ Group fitness classes that involve jumping and running.

BEFORE COMMENCING YOUR EXERCISE PROGRAM . . .

If you have health problems, or if you have not exercised previously or if you are very unfit, *always check with your doctor before commencing an exercise program.* Start your exercise program slowly if you are unaccustomed to exercising, and progress gradually as your strength and fitness improve.

HOW SHOULD YOU EXERCISE FOR GOOD HEALTH?

Now that you know the type of exercise that is best for your body, you also need to know just how much and how hard you need to exercise to get your body fit and healthy. The following official guidelines on exercising for optimal health have been established by the American College of Sports Medicine and the American Heart Association.[5]

EXERCISE GUIDELINES FOR HEALTHY, ACTIVE INDIVIDUALS AGED 18–65 YEARS OLD

For aerobic fitness your exercise program should involve:

- ♀ at least 5 days of aerobic fitness activities per week
- ♀ 30 minutes of continuous exercise or intermittent bouts of at least 10 minutes each (at least 2.5 hrs/week)
- ♀ moderate intensity ...

OR

- ♀ at least 3 days of aerobic fitness exercise per week
- ♀ 20-minute sessions
- ♀ vigorous intensity.

How intensely are you exercising[6]?

Use the following scale to measure your exercise intensity.

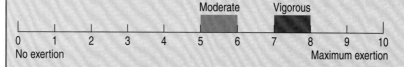

Moderate exercise should feel as though you are working at 5–6 out of 10. Moderately intense exercise noticeably raises your heart and breathing rate (but allows you to carry on a conversation).

Vigorous exercise should feel as though you are working at 7–8 out of 10. Vigorous-intensity exercise causes a substantial increase in your heart rate and rapid breathing.

Improve your fitness and lose your fat 41

EXERCISE GUIDELINES FOR INDIVIDUALS AGED OVER 65 YEARS OR ADULTS 50–64 WITH CHRONIC CONDITIONS REQUIRING REGULAR MEDICAL TREATMENT[6]

Develop a physical activity plan with a health professional to identify and manage your needs and risks.

AND

Follow the same exercise prescription listed above for 18–65-year-olds.

HOW SHOULD YOU MAINTAIN YOUR FITNESS?

In order to maintain your aerobic fitness, you must continue regular exercise on an ongoing basis. If you cease exercise altogether, your fitness will decline back to the level it was before you started exercising.

To get myself fit again I needed to start looking after myself. I started to get honest with myself about what I was putting into my mouth. I tried to cut down on how much I was eating (especially fat) and how much alcohol I was drinking. I was referred to a physio who treated my back and my back pain started to settle down a little bit.

I started to exercise and this helped me a lot. I was taught about my core muscles and how to exercise them properly. I had never done pelvic floor exercises before but even after a couple of weeks of doing them I noticed that I was feeling drier. I started walking for about half an hour every morning. I also started going to aqua classes and doing some cycling and walking in the pool. On the weekends my husband and I returned to bushwalking which we hadn't done for years. As I exercised and started to lose weight, I felt as though I had more energy to do more, and I wanted to do more because I wasn't so damp all the time. In the last three months I have lost 5 kg and I can fit into my clothes again. I definitely feel a lot better, happier and I am sleeping better too. I now know that exercise helps me to feel good and get the most out of my life.

Linda

WEIGHT LOSS AND YOUR PELVIC FLOOR

If you are carrying a little too much weight, you have the capacity to do your pelvic floor a big favour by losing some kilos. If you can reduce your weight even a little, you will reduce the load your pelvic floor has to carry around all day. This may help to reduce your pelvic floor symptoms if you already have them, and decrease the likelihood of pelvic floor problems occurring or worsening in the future. If you are overweight, reducing your weight will also undoubtedly help you to decrease many of the potentially negative effects of menopause upon your body—so it's really worth making the effort to knock off those extra kilos!

> **Weight loss tip**
> Always check with your general practitioner before commencing a weight loss program.

THE WINNING WEIGHT LOSS COMBINATION = SENSIBLE DIET + EFFECTIVE EXERCISE

Many of us know how disheartening trying to lose weight can be, especially when results are slow to appear. The first step you will need to make is to reduce your overall calorie intake. Then if you can combine your reduced energy intake with an increase in the energy you use up, you will have a winning combination for weight loss. Exercise alone will only result in modest weight loss. Sometimes moving more if you have a pelvic floor problem is easier said than done. If moving makes you leak or feel uncomfortable, you will obviously feel less inclined to move. The following guidelines are designed to help you towards your goal of a healthier body.

> **Weight loss tip**
> Try to create an energy deficit of 500–1000 calories/day through a combination of exercise and reduced energy intake. Based upon this deficit, a goal of 0.5–0.9 kg/week weight loss is realistic.[7]

HOW SHOULD YOU EXERCISE TO LOSE WEIGHT?

You have already read that you need to aim for 30 minutes of moderate exercise 5 days per week for your general health. The more exercise you perform every week, the more likely you are to lose weight and keep it off. Official recommendations suggest that for permanent weight loss, ideally you should build up the amount of moderate-intensity aerobic exercise you do up to 3.3–5 hours per week.[7] This may seem like a lot of aerobic exercise for some of us. If you are not one for exercising for lengthy periods of time, you may find that commencing with 10–15 minute bouts of exercise will help you to start to incorporate more exercise into your life.

HOW TO BURN MORE FAT WITH EXERCISE

Increase the time you spend exercising

Increase the amount of time you spend performing moderately intense aerobic exercise every week. You may find that you can gradually increase the length of your exercise sessions as your strength and endurance increase. Training your pelvic floor and deep abdominal muscles may also increase your capacity to exercise for longer by reducing your symptoms. If longer sessions are not manageable because of time or discomfort, try to include more short exercise sessions into your weekly routine. The more exercise you can manage to do in total, the more energy your body will use up during each session and long after you finish exercising.

Choose low-impact aerobic exercise

Choose from the low-impact exercises listed in this chapter. If you leak when you walk, you may find whole-body–supported exercise such as stationary cycling has the least effect upon your symptoms. Cycling is a great way to burn energy and minimize your symptoms. Why not hire an exercise bike? Or pick up a second-hand exercise bike if your finances are limited.

Use more muscle

The most effective type of exercise for burning fat is exercise that involves the most muscle. Your large muscles store and burn the most energy. In order to replenish their energy stores, these muscles will continue to burn fat long after you finish exercising. Choose exercise that uses large muscles such as your leg muscles, e.g. cycling and walking. Increase the energy you use up by swinging your arms as you walk.

Mix up your workouts

Have you ever been frustrated by doing the same exercise routine day in, day out, and never losing any weight? Your muscles become very efficient at using energy if you exercise the same way every time. Make your muscles use more energy by varying your aerobic exercise routine. Choose different types of low-impact exercise, vary the order and the time you spend on different exercises as often as you can—every time you exercise if possible.

Increase your incidental exercise

Seize every opportunity to incorporate extra exercise into your normal activities. Simple strategies such as choosing the stairs instead of the lift, or parking your car to allow you a short brisk walk to your destination, will improve your ability to manage your weight.

Perform strength exercises regularly

Hormonal changes associated with menopause cause your body to lose muscle. Resistance or strength training will not give you a large, bulky body; in fact quite the reverse, as muscle tissue is lean and it uses up energy. Resistance training improves the strength and endurance of your muscles. A good resistance-training program will help you to move with less effort and encourage you to move more and burn more energy. Appropriate resistance-training exercises are detailed in Chapter 6.

Key points to improving your fitness and staying power

- Aerobic exercise increases your stamina and cardiovascular fitness.
- Appropriate aerobic exercise can improve your mind and body.
- Perform low-impact aerobic exercise to protect your pelvic floor.
- To protect your pelvic floor, avoid high-impact exercise involving both feet off the ground surface, or stepping heavily.
- If you are 18–65 years old and healthy, promote your aerobic fitness with:
  - moderate-intensity exercise for at least 30 minutes, 5 days per week; OR
  - vigorous exercise for at least 20 minutes, 3 days per week.
- If you are over 65 years old or 50 to 64 with a chronic condition, you should develop an exercise plan with a health professional.
- Your aerobic fitness gains will be lost without regular ongoing exercise.
- Combine sensible diet and effective exercise to lose body fat.
- Aim for an energy deficit of 500–1000 calories/day and realistic weight loss of 0.5–0.9 kg/week.
- To burn fat when you exercise:
  - gradually increase the duration of your aerobic workouts;
  - choose a variety of low-impact exercises;
  - mix up your aerobic workouts;
  - increase your incidental exercise; and
  - perform strength-training exercises.
- To lose body fat and keep it off, aim for 3.3–5 hrs/week of moderate-intensity exercise.

6 Get your body strong—active workouts

Women are now recognizing the enormous benefits of resistance training, particularly in overcoming the effects of aging (and gravity)! Resistance training is an excellent form of exercise to help you stay healthy and active. It specifically addresses some of the changes to your body associated with menopause and growing older. Strength training can help you to prevent disease and injury, manage your weight, stay strong and toned, and feel confident and capable of easily doing the activities you want to do every day. So what are you waiting for?

> *I am 45 years old and I was recently diagnosed with a vaginal prolapse. My specialist has told me to avoid heavy lifting but my GP has also told me I need to do some strength exercises because my bone density is already decreased. My mum had terrible fractures in her spine from her osteoporosis and she lived with constant back pain. I am really anxious about what I should do and frustrated as I like to exercise—it makes me feel good about myself and helps me cope with stress. Now every time I try to do anything I can feel a horrible bulging for the rest of the day. Until recently I was going to the gym and doing weights but now I've stopped. I feel like my body is falling apart and I'm scared to do anything.*
>
> Susan

ARE YOU CONFUSED ABOUT HOW TO SAFELY IMPROVE YOUR STRENGTH?

If you are a woman with pelvic floor problems, you may be terrified of muscle-strength training for fear of leakage or further pelvic floor injury. You can take heart in knowing that you can perform strength-training exercises. The key is knowing just what exercises you can do and how to do them safely. In fact, strength training your whole body may even help you to take a load off your pelvic floor during your daily activities.

WHAT IS RESISTANCE TRAINING?

Resistance or strength training involves using your muscles against a load or force to make them stronger. Different types of resistance training include free weights, weight machines, water resistance, exercise tubing and using your own body weight. Remember that muscle is lean tissue and that you will not develop large, bulky muscles from resistance training. You are actually more likely to feel trim and toned as a result of this type of exercise.

> *Before I started strength training I felt as though my body was ageing fast. Since I started doing my strength exercises I've noticed a big difference in myself. I am much stronger and I have much more energy. I am able to do things that were becoming difficult for me like getting up off the ground. I feel much more confident, and I am much more active, so it has certainly improved me.*

Pat, age 62

HOW RESISTANCE TRAINING CAN HELP YOU

Some of the potential benefits for you and your body include:

- ♀ Increasing your strength and endurance
- ♀ Increasing your lean muscle and decreasing your body fat
- ♀ Increasing your bone density and preventing osteoporosis
- ♀ Preventing or managing diseases and conditions such as diabetes, cardiovascular problems and lower back pain
- ♀ Improving your ability to move, and reducing your likelihood of falls
- ♀ Reducing your stress levels
- ♀ Improving your self-confidence

OSTEOPOROSIS AND YOUR PELVIC FLOOR

Bone loss starts in your mid-forties and proceeds rapidly at the onset of menopause. Osteoporosis can have a negative effect on your continence. Some medications for osteoporosis can cause constipation and straining, thereby affecting your pelvic floor. Spinal fractures can exacerbate pelvic floor problems by causing a slumped-forward posture and increasing pressure in your abdomen. If your movement is affected by an osteoporosis-related fracture, it can become very difficult to reach the toilet in time.

Exercise is a major factor in preventing and managing osteoporosis. If you restrict your physical activity to prevent leakage, your likelihood of falling and fracturing a bone may increase as a result of your poor physical condition. One of the most important things you can do to minimize bone loss is to incorporate appropriate exercise into your regular routine.

There are two types of exercise important to keep your bones strong:

1. **Weight-bearing exercise**—exercise which involves carrying your weight through your feet.
2. **Resistance exercise**—exercise which involves moving your muscles against a load.

If you have pelvic floor problems you will realize that both the above types of exercise can potentially aggravate your condition. This means you need to be clever about the way you exercise. Bone-Fit for Beginners[8] is a physiotherapist-designed home exercise DVD specifically designed to teach you how to correctly perform resistance exercises for strong muscles and bones, with strength exercises that place minimal strain upon your pelvic floor.

PROCEED WITH CAUTION!

Before you go rushing off to the nearest gym, beware, as resistance training has the potential to have an adverse effect upon your pelvic floor. *In particular, you need to pay attention to the type of resistance exercises you perform, the heaviness of the load, and your technique in performing these exercises.* It is advisable to have a qualified instructor, exercise professional or physiotherapist show you how to safely use strength-training equipment; and always employ the following "Pelvic Floor Protection Principles" for safe strengthening.

PELVIC FLOOR PROTECTION PRINCIPLES

1. **Avoid heavy lifting**

   Keep your weights within a manageable range. Never lift heavy weights that make you strain or inclined to hold your breath. If you have pelvic floor problems, you must keep your resistance to a minimum until your pelvic floor muscle condition has improved. Avoid lifting weights from ground level if possible; instead, aim to lift from waist height.

2. **Use your pelvic floor muscles**

   Activate your pelvic floor muscles prior to and during your resistance exercises. The goal is for your pelvic floor to be working immediately before and as you lift/lower/push or pull any load.

3. **Lift with good posture**

   Maintain the normal inward curve in your lower back during every lift/lower/push/pull exercise you do, regardless of whether you are sitting, standing or lying on your back. This will promote the protective activity of your supportive deep abdominal and pelvic floor muscles and discourage the activity of your strong outer abdominal muscles.

4. **Exhale with every effort**

   Never hold your breath or pull your stomach in strongly during your exercise as this increases the downward pressure on your pelvic floor. Breathe out with every effort, whether it is a lift, push or pull, to reduce the likelihood of straining your pelvic floor.

5. **Choose supported positions**

   Your pelvic floor will be under less strain if you perform your resistance exercises sitting or lying down wherever possible. Sitting on an exercise ball is an excellent option while you perform your strength exercises. It will promote the activity of your deep abdominal muscles, support your pelvic floor, decrease the likelihood of symptoms as you exercise, and make it easier to feel your pelvic floor muscles working.

6. **Keep your feet close together**

   You will find it easier to activate your pelvic floor muscles when your feet are close together and your pelvic floor openings are less exposed. If you are performing a standing resistance exercise, try to keep your feet no wider than hip width apart rather than wide-leg standing positions. Hip width means that your knees should be approximately fist width apart.

7. **Strengthen gradually**

   Start using very light resistance and pay attention to performing the exercise correctly to reduce your risk of injury. Gradually increase your load when you are very confident of your technique and when you have good pelvic floor and abdominal muscle control.

8. **Take care when fatigued or injured**

   When you are very tired, unwell or have lower back pain, your pelvic floor and deep abdominal muscles may not work as effectively and you will be more prone to symptoms and injury. Take a break and return to resistance training when you have recovered.

9. **Rest between sets**

   Rest for a couple of minutes between each set of exercises you perform. This gives your muscles (including your pelvic floor muscles) time to recover before your next lift.

10. **Avoid aggravating exercises and machines**

    Listen to your body when exercising. If your symptoms are worse with a specific exercise, modify that exercise or leave it out of your program and perform another exercise to strengthen the same area. Specific exercises and machines to avoid are detailed in Chapter 7.

I had always enjoyed going to the gym before my prolapse got worse. I worked with a personal trainer but now when I look back I realize that what I was doing was causing me more harm than good. I ended up needing surgery for my prolapse and then after that I put on a lot of weight as I was too afraid to do anything. I became quite depressed. I was sent to a physio who took me through a program of exercises and I learnt the correct techniques to allow me to strength train again. I have now been going back to the gym for two months and exercising safely. I realize I don't need to lift heavy weights to get results. I am feeling stronger, fitter and much happier and looking forward to staying active in the future.

Debbie, age 48

SUITABLE STRENGTH-TRAINING EXERCISES

You can perform the following whole-body strength exercises with confidence that you are improving your strength AND protecting your pelvic floor as you do so. Remember to follow the "Pelvic Floor Protection Principles" already outlined, particularly if you have or are at risk of pelvic floor problems. You can choose strength exercises from the following list. Variations are also provided for you to change your program. You can perform the following exercises either at home or in the gym.

LEG STRENGTH EXERCISES

Narrow Leg Squats

Squats are a great exercise for strengthening your thighs and buttocks. This exercise will also improve the ease of your everyday activities.

- ♀ Start with your back towards a wall, and place your exercise ball in the curve of your lower back.
- ♀ Walk your feet out in front of your body. To protect your knees, make sure you can see your toes in front of your knees throughout your entire squat.
- ♀ Lift your chest and lengthen your spine.

Inside Out

- ♀ Squeeze and lift your pelvic floor muscles.

- ♀ Bend your knees and lower your buttocks down towards the ground, ensuring that your buttocks remain above the height of your knees at the deepest part of your squat, as shown in Figure 6.1.

- ♀ Avoid deep squats, particularly if you are prone to knee pain.

- ♀ Maintain your pelvic floor muscle contraction as you push through your heels and straighten your legs to return back up to your starting position.

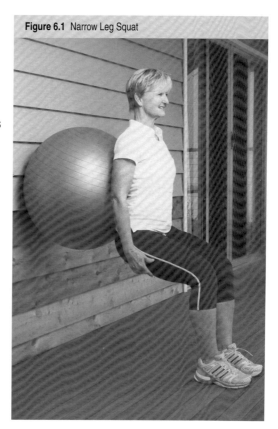

Figure 6.1 Narrow Leg Squat

| Pelvic floor tips | Keep your feet and knees approximately hip width apart throughout and breathe out during your squat. |

Squat variations include:

- ♀ Squat and reach your arms forward as you bend your knees.
- ♀ Hold a set of dumbbells on your hips.
- ♀ Weighted "Squat and Bend" exercise, as outlined in Chapter 4.

Forward Lunge

This exercise will strengthen and tone your thighs and your buttocks.

- Start with your legs in a long-stride position.
- Throughout the entire exercise, make sure that your front knee remains directly above your front ankle and not forward over your toes. Avoid deep lunges especially if you are prone to knee pain.
- Activate your pelvic floor muscles before and as you move your body.
- Bend both of your knees, lowering your back knee down towards the ground as shown in Figure 6.2.
- Raise your body back up to your starting position.

Suitable lunge variations include:

- Back-to-ball wall lunge.
- Dumbbell lunge.
- Step forward/backward lunge.
- Travelling lunge.

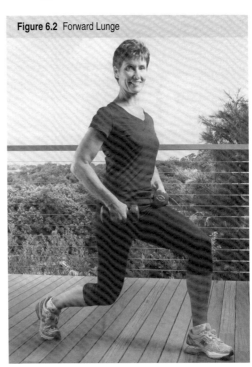

Figure 6.2 Forward Lunge

Pelvic floor tip Breathe out as you lift your body back to your starting position.

Floor Bridge

Bridging will promote the strength of the back of your thighs, buttocks and your lower back.

- ♀ Start by lying on your back with your heels close to your buttocks and your weights across the front of your hips.
- ♀ If you are using weights, rest them comfortably across the front of your hips as shown in Figure 6.3.
- ♀ Activate your pelvic floor muscles before and as you raise your body.
- ♀ Push down through your heels and lift your buttocks off the ground, squeezing your buttocks together and lifting your body as shown in Figure 6.3.
- ♀ Gently lower your body back down to the ground.

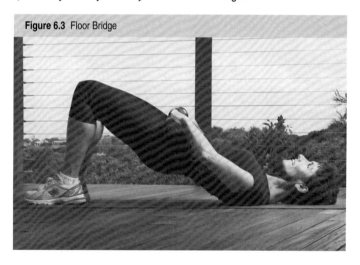

Figure 6.3 Floor Bridge

Hip strength variation includes:
- ♀ Floor ball bridge with your feet resting on an exercise ball.

Pelvic floor tip — Breathe out as you raise your buttocks off the ground.

Get your body strong—active workouts 55

Calf Raises

Calf raises will improve your calf strength and improve your balance.

- Stand and lightly hold onto a bench if your balance is decreased.
- Lift your heels off the ground as shown in Figure 6.4.
- Lower your body back down to your starting position.

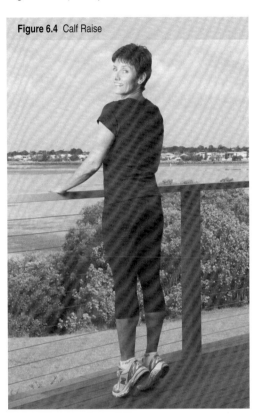

Figure 6.4 Calf Raise

> Suitable calf strength variations include:
> - Calf raise holding dumbbells.
> - Single-leg calf raise.

Pelvic floor tip — Practice keeping your pelvic floor muscles active during this exercise.

BACK STRENGTH EXERCISES

Back strengthening is very useful to improve your posture for everyday activities. Improving your posture will also help to improve your deep abdominal and pelvic floor muscle control.

Low Dumbbell Row

This is a particularly good exercise to strengthen the postural muscles between your shoulder blades and your spine. It will also help you to perform your everyday pulling and lifting activities.

- ♀ Start by leaning your upper body forward and supported by your left hand and left knee on the seat of a chair or on an exercise ball.
- ♀ Keep your right knee slightly bent to protect your spine.
- ♀ Hold a dumbbell in your right hand with your right arm extended next to your right thigh.
- ♀ Tuck your chin towards your chest to protect your neck.
- ♀ Activate your pelvic floor muscles before and as you lift your dumbbell.
- ♀ Pull your right arm back and up, by bending your right elbow towards the ceiling as shown in Figure 6.5.

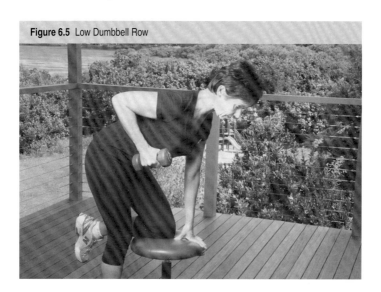

Figure 6.5 Low Dumbbell Row

- ♀ Feel your right shoulder blade move inwards towards your spine as you raise your right elbow.
- ♀ Slowly lower your right arm back to your starting position.
- ♀ Relax your pelvic floor muscles.
- ♀ Repeat the same exercise with your left arm.

Pelvic floor tips Maintain the curve in your lower back throughout this exercise and exhale as you raise your dumbbell. Try to keep your pelvic floor muscles activated for an entire set of exercises. If you cannot manage this, rest briefly and then start again.

Back-strength variations include:

- ♀ Low dumbbell row, lying forward over an exercise ball.
- ♀ Wide dumbbell row with your elbow held perpendicular to your body and in line with your shoulder as you raise and lower your dumbbell.

CHEST STRENGTH EXERCISES

The following exercises will help you to strengthen the muscles of your chest and the front of your shoulders.

Flat Dumbbell Press

This exercise will help you to strengthen the chest and shoulder muscles that you use in everyday pushing activities.

- ♀ Lie on your back with your knees bent.
- ♀ Squeeze and lift your pelvic floor muscles.
- ♀ Hold a dumbbell in each hand and extend your arms towards the ceiling to position the dumbbells directly above your chest with your palms facing the direction of your feet, as shown in Figure 6.6.
- ♀ Slowly lower your dumbbells directly down to your shoulders, keeping your elbows out in line with your shoulders and your palms facing your feet. Your elbows should be lowered so that they are perpendicular to your body.
- ♀ Raise the dumbbells back to your starting position.
- ♀ Relax your pelvic floor muscles when finished.

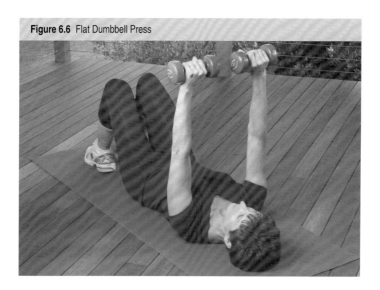

Figure 6.6 Flat Dumbbell Press

Pelvic floor tips

Maintain your inward lower back curve and never strain when performing chest exercises. Breathe out as you raise your dumbbells to the ceiling. Decrease potential strain on your pelvic floor by raising only one dumbbell at a time. Try to keep your pelvic floor muscles active whilst exercising. If they fatigue, stop and rest briefly then start again.

Chest strength variations include:

- ♀ Flat dumbbell press, lying on a bench or an exercise ball.
- ♀ Inclined dumbbell press, lying on an inclined bench.
- ♀ Lying dumbbell fly.

SHOULDER AND ARM STRENGTH EXERCISES

If your upper body is strong for lifting, you may be less likely to strain when you lift during your everyday activities. The following exercises will improve your ability to perform your everyday lifting activities in addition to toning your shoulders and arms.

Rotator Cuff

This is a great exercise to strengthen your shoulders and improve your posture.

- ♀ Start by sitting tall with good posture on a chair or an exercise ball.
- ♀ Hold your bent elbows beside your body, and face your palms and dumbbells towards each other.
- ♀ Squeeze and lift your pelvic floor muscles before and as you move your dumbbells.
- ♀ Keep your upper arms in contact with your sides throughout the entire exercise as you move your dumbbells backwards, as shown in Figure 6.7.
- ♀ Move your dumbbells back to your starting position.
- ♀ Relax your pelvic floor muscles when you have completed your set of exercises.

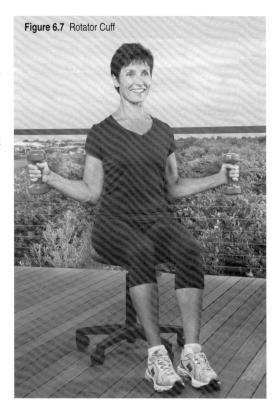

Figure 6.7 Rotator Cuff

Bicep Curl (front of upper arm)

Bicep curls will make you strong for lifting and tone your upper arms.

- ♀ Start sitting tall with good posture on a chair or exercise ball.
- ♀ Grasp your dumbbells with your arms extended by your sides.
- ♀ Squeeze and lift your pelvic floor muscles.
- ♀ Lift your left dumbbell towards your left shoulder by bending that elbow, as shown in Figure 6.8.
- ♀ Slowly lower your dumbbell back to your starting position.
- ♀ Relax your pelvic floor muscles when you have completed your set of exercises.
- ♀ Repeat this exercise with your left arm.

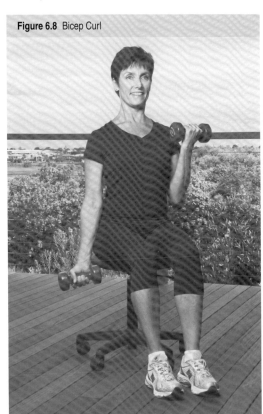

Figure 6.8 Bicep Curl

Shoulder strength variation includes:

- ♀ Dumbbell lateral raise.
- ♀ Upright dumbbell row.

Inside Out

Tricep Press Back (back of upper arm)

Tricep exercises will strengthen and tone the back of your upper arms.

- ♀ Start sitting on a chair or exercise ball.
- ♀ Grasp your dumbbell in your right hand.
- ♀ Lean forward and support your upper body with your left forearm resting on your thighs.
- ♀ Tuck your right elbow and upper arm into the right side of your body.
- ♀ Straighten your right elbow and press your dumbbell backwards keeping this elbow held high, as shown in Figure 6.9.
- ♀ Bend your elbow to lower the dumbbell back to your starting position.
- ♀ Keep your gaze directed to your feet to protect your neck throughout this exercise.
- ♀ Repeat this exercise with your left arm.

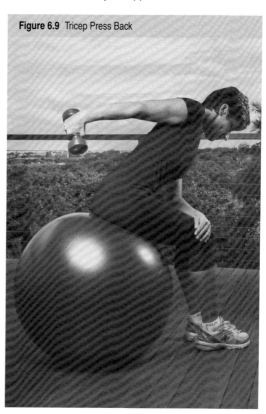

Figure 6.9 Tricep Press Back

Pelvic floor tips

Protect your pelvic floor by doing these exercises in supported positions. Decrease the load on your pelvic floor by moving one dumbbell at a time. Breathe out as you raise your dumbbell.

HOW MUCH RESISTANCE TRAINING SHOULD YOU DO?

For improved strength and well-being you should follow the resistance training guidelines below, as set out by the American College of Sports Medicine.[9]

RESISTANCE TRAINING GUIDELINES FOR HEALTHY WOMEN 18–65 YEARS OLD

- ♀ Perform resistance exercise on at least 2 alternate days per week.
- ♀ Choose 8–10 strength exercises for the major muscle groups.
- ♀ Perform a minimum of 8–12 repetitions (1 set) of each strength exercise.
- ♀ Perform between 1–3 sets of repetitions of each strength exercise.
- ♀ Progressively increase your resistance as your strength improves.

RESISTANCE TRAINING GUIDELINES FOR WOMEN OVER 65 YEARS OR 50–64 YEARS WITH CHRONIC CONDITIONS

- ♀ Perform resistance exercise on at least 2–3 alternate days per week.
- ♀ Choose 10 strength exercises for the major muscle groups.
- ♀ Perform 10–15 repetitions of each strength exercise.

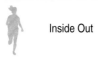

Key points for getting your body strong

- Resistance training involves strengthening your muscles by using them against a load or force.
- Strength exercise will provide you with many health benefits.
- You need to be cautious about strength exercises in order to protect your pelvic floor.
- Always use the "Pelvic Floor Protection Principles" to minimize pelvic floor strain when performing strength exercises.
- Choose strength-training exercises that will place minimal strain on your pelvic floor.
- Healthy women 18–65 years old should perform strength exercises on 2–3 alternate days per week with 1–3 sets of 8–12 repetitions using the major muscle groups to keep strong and healthy.
- Suitable strength exercises include:

  Narrow Leg Squats   Flat Dumbbell Press
  Forward Lunge   Rotator Cuff
  Floor Bridge   Bicep Curl
  Calf Raises   Tricep Press Back
  Low Dumbbell Row

7 Gym and equipment exercises exposed!

More and more women are launching themselves into the gym or organized circuit training classes in order to stay fit, strong and healthy. This chapter is designed to help you confidently choose the right strength exercises for your pelvic floor when you are at the gym and when using exercise equipment. Remember that having read this book you may actually be better informed about the effect of particular exercises on your pelvic floor than your instructor. Gym instructors usually have great intentions and know how to get your body fit; however, they may not understand the effect of some of their exercises on your pelvic floor.

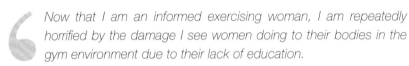

Now that I am an informed exercising woman, I am repeatedly horrified by the damage I see women doing to their bodies in the gym environment due to their lack of education.

After learning the "right way" to move and exercise as a woman and how to protect and strengthen the areas that hold me stable and in control, for the past year I have been able to exercise at a level far greater than I would have ever thought I was capable of. My muscle strength has improved beyond what I would have considered possible in the past. When sharing my success with my girlfriends, I am amazed how many women suffer these symptoms, with no idea that their current exercise regimes are worsening, if not causing their problems, or that they can easily and effectively improve or correct the damage they are doing. I am thrilled to know that now as I approach menopause and beyond I am armed with knowledge and techniques that will keep me strong, stable and my insides healthy.

Leanne, age 42

STRENGTH TRAINING EQUIPMENT TO USE WITH CONFIDENCE

You can perform the following equipment-based exercises comfortable in the knowledge that they are the most appropriate for minimizing strain upon your pelvic floor. Remember to adhere to the "Pelvic Floor Protection Principles" outlined in Chapter 6. The following list of exercises is designed for you to take along to your fitness center. You may need to ask a qualified instructor to demonstrate the correct use of any equipment you are unsure about.

Appropriate equipment-based exercises:

- ♀ Leg extension
- ♀ Prone leg curl
- ♀ Seated leg curl
- ♀ Smith machine-assisted lunges
- ♀ Seated calf raise
- ♀ Seated row
- ♀ Smith machine-assisted chest press
- ♀ Pec deck
- ♀ Seated shoulder press
- ♀ Seated military press
- ♀ Seated preacher curl using EZ-curl bar
- ♀ Triceps push-down machine (sit on an exercise ball)

Pelvic floor tip — Always keep your weights within a manageable range and NEVER STRAIN.

My first baby was a big boy (9 lb 5 oz). He was a forceps delivery. My body has never been the same since. I have always loved exercising, it makes me feel good. Recently I started to notice a bulging heavy feeling in my vagina especially after the gym and I was absolutely devastated when my GP told me that that I had a prolapse and that I had to stop heavy exercise. I cried all the way home. I was so humiliated. I had no idea that childbirth and the wrong kind of exercise could affect me this way.

Carol, age 47

GYM EXERCISES TO AVOID

If you already have or are at risk of pelvic floor problems, you should try to avoid any exercise with the potential to strain your pelvic floor. The following exercises all have the potential to increase the downward pressure upon your pelvic floor and are best avoided for this reason:

- ♀ Abdominal strength machines (detailed next in this chapter)
- ♀ Leg press machine
- ♀ Dead lifts
- ♀ Men's push-ups
- ♀ Chin-ups
- ♀ Chest dips
- ♀ Wide-leg squats
- ♀ Jump squats
- ♀ Side lunges
- ♀ High bench step-up/step-down
- ♀ Triceps dips with both feet off the ground
- ♀ Lat pull-down with heavy weight

ABDOMINAL EXERCISES TO AVOID

If you have pelvic floor problems or if you are at risk of them, you need to stop exercising your strong outer abdominal muscles with exercises like sit-ups. Your outer abdominal muscles can greatly increase the downward pressure on your pelvic floor. If you exercise these muscles, you will make them stronger and better at pushing your pelvic floor downwards. Repeatedly exercising them may increase your incontinence and prolapse symptoms. Using ultrasound to study bladder movement, it has been observed that when women with pelvic floor problems performed abdominal curls, their bladders were forced downwards.[10]

Sit-ups are not the only exercises designed to strengthen your outer abdominals. There are many other exercises and machines designed to do this and some are commonly used in women's circuit classes. Do your pelvic floor a favour and avoid these exercises if you have or are at risk of pelvic floor problems:

- ♀ Abdominal curl/crunch
- ♀ Abdominal curl machine
- ♀ Oblique sit-ups
- ♀ Oblique machine
- ♀ Ball sit-ups
- ♀ Twisting crunch
- ♀ Incline sit-ups
- ♀ Rope crunch
- ♀ Double leg raise
- ♀ Hanging knee raise
- ♀ Ball-between-leg lifts
- ♀ Bicycle legs

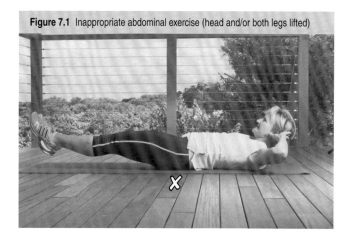

Figure 7.1 Inappropriate abdominal exercise (head and/or both legs lifted)

> **Pelvic floor tip**
>
> Your outer abdominal muscles are exercised strongly when you perform any exercises that involve either lifting your head and upper body off the ground and/or raising both your legs off the ground at the same time. Avoid any exercise with your head and shoulders lifted and/or both legs raised off the ground at once, as shown in Figure 7.1. This exercise has been shown to increase pressure within the abdomen and requires very strong pelvic floor muscle activity to counteract this pressure, even in women without pelvic floor dysfunction.[11]

ABDOMINAL EXERCISES REQUIRING YOUR CAUTION

Popular gym exercises such as hover, plank and push-up will not specifically strengthen your pelvic floor. These exercises will strengthen your strong, outer abdominal muscles. Perform these exercises with caution and only if you are not at risk of pelvic floor dysfunction. Cease these exercises if they cause you any symptoms.

If you really feel you must do these exercises, make them a little kinder to your pelvic floor by performing them while supporting your weight through your knees rather than through your feet, as shown in the modified hover exercise in Figure 7.2.

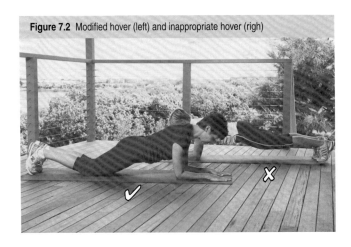

Figure 7.2 Modified hover (left) and inappropriate hover (righ)

Key points for gym and equipment exercise

- ♀ Use exercise equipment that allows you to protect your pelvic floor.
- ♀ Some popular gym and circuit equipment can increase your symptoms and potentially strain your pelvic floor.
- ♀ Use caution when exercising in a gym and when using exercise equipment.
- ♀ Some popular abdominal strength exercises have the potential to damage your pelvic floor and worsen your symptoms.
- ♀ Keep your weights within a manageable range and never strain.
- ♀ Choose exercise equipment that supports your body where possible.
- ♀ Adhere to the "Pelvic Floor Protection Principles" when using strength training equipment.
- ♀ If your pelvic floor muscles are weak or if you are at increased risk of pelvic floor dysfunction, avoid exercises and equipment that strengthen your outer abdominal muscles.

8 Exercise classes and your insides

Group exercise can be a great fun way to exercise. Exercise classes can provide you with motivation and instruction to help you improve your health. Sometimes it is difficult to know whether a particular exercise class or specific exercises within a class have the potential to strain your pelvic floor or cause you embarrassing symptoms. You will need to consider the potential effect of the exercises and the class situation upon your body. How much does your instructor know about your pelvic floor and the exercises you need to avoid? Is the class low impact? Does the class include exercises that may aggravate your condition?

If you are concerned about particular exercises, have a quiet word with your instructor prior to the class and explain that there may be some exercises that you may not be able to perform during the class for health reasons. Exercising in a group may make you feel more compelled to do an exercise that you know you should avoid. Be sure to listen to your body, and exercise only at your own level of personal comfort and ability.

> *I realized some of the cause of my condition was a little extra weight that I carried and a lack of muscle strength. So I knew WHAT I needed to change to improve my level of comfort but had limited instruction as to HOW to change it. In an attempt to "get fit and strong" I tried various different types of exercise from brisk walking/jogging, aerobic classes, pump classes and stationary machines at the gym. To my frustration, I would find that this would always result in exacerbating my condition. I then became apprehensive about resuming exercise and my motivation was lower with each failed attempt.*

Judy, age 49

BEST GROUP EXERCISE CLASSES FOR YOUR PELVIC FLOOR

The following group exercise classes are low impact and are therefore best suited to protecting your pelvic floor. Remember that some specific exercises in some of these classes may increase the load on your pelvic floor, so try to avoid these exercises or modify them whenever you can. Read the following tips to help you to protect your pelvic floor when you participate in these particular classes.

AQUA AEROBICS OR WATER FITNESS CLASSES

Aqua classes involve water-based exercise. This type of exercise supports your body weight and absorbs shock, thereby reducing the impact upon your pelvic floor and the stress upon your joints. Exercising in water may enhance your muscle strength and endurance, aerobic fitness, flexibility and balance. Deeper water will lessen the load upon your pelvic floor.

Aqua tips

- ♀ If the water is lower than your chest level, try to avoid running and jumping. Instead keep these exercises low impact with fast walking, marching on the spot or side-stepping.
- ♀ Avoid abdominal exercises that may take the form of cycling your legs whilst lying on your back and abdominal crunch-style exercises such as pulling both knees to your chest at the same time.

GROUP CYCLE OR "SPIN" CLASSES

Cycle classes are low impact and involve riding a stationary bike with adjustable leg resistance. Cycle classes can improve your aerobic fitness and allow you to exercise at a vigorous intensity with minimal compromise to your pelvic floor. Cycling will also increase your leg strength.

Cycle tips	♀ Avoid using heavy resistance through your legs. ♀ Stay seated if the class includes out-of-the-seat/saddle-climbing tracks. ♀ Activate your deep abdominal muscles gently, not forcefully, when leaning forward and riding your bike.

YOGA

There are many types of yoga that incorporate physical exercise as a part of achieving the yoga goal of mind and body union. Yoga classes involve a series of exercises or postures that have potential physical benefits for your strength, flexibility, posture and breathing awareness.

Yoga tips	♀ Make sure you use appropriate abdominal muscle activation, posture and breathing technique during yoga postures. ♀ Avoid exercises involving both legs raised together off the ground, such as "Double Leg Lift" and "Boat Pose", and modify these by keeping your head down on the ground and raising only one leg at a time. ♀ Modify the "Plank" position so that you support your body weight through your knees rather than through your feet, as illustrated in exercise modification in Figure 7.2. ♀ Avoid wide-leg standing poses that involve bending forwards with your legs wide apart, such as "Legs Wide Forward Bend". ♀ Avoid wide, deep, squat positions like "Garland Pose". ♀ Avoid maintained wide-leg poses and instead hold your poses in stride position. ♀ Avoid poses that involve weight bearing entirely through your upper body.

EXERCISE BALL OR SWISS BALL CLASSES

Exercise ball classes use large, inflatable balls for supported exercises in upright and lying positions. These classes may also incorporate hand weights for muscle strengthening. Exercise ball classes have potential benefits for your posture, muscle strength, deep abdominal control, balance and flexibility.

Exercise ball tips

- ♀ Avoid exercises on the ball that use your outer abdominal muscles, e.g. sit-ups, push-ups, hovers, and lifting the ball off the ground with it placed between your legs.

- ♀ Avoid higher-impact exercises that involve jumping up and down on the ball.

- ♀ You will get the most benefit out of exercise ball classes by ensuring your good posture and deep abdominal muscle control throughout.

DANCE CLASSES

Low-impact dance classes such as ballroom, country and western, Latin-American and belly dancing are all suitable forms of group exercise that will usually place minimal stress upon your pelvic floor. Dance classes will potentially benefit your aerobic fitness, balance and flexibility.

TAI CHI

Tai Chi is a system of slow-flowing, standing body postures and coordinated movements based upon traditional Chinese martial arts. Tai Chi will potentially benefit your balance, flexibility, cardiorespiratory function and bone density. Most Tai Chi exercises will place minimal pressure upon your pelvic floor.

EXERCISE CLASSES THAT MAY *NOT* BE SUITED TO YOUR PELVIC FLOOR

The following classes all have potential benefits for your general health; however, some exercises that may be in these classes also have the potential to increase the load upon your pelvic floor. If you already have or are at increased risk of pelvic floor problems, participate in these classes with caution and modify those exercises with the potential to cause you injury or symptoms. If you are unable to avoid potentially dangerous exercises in these classes, choose an alternative class. If you find any of the following classes exacerbate your symptoms, avoid them at least until your pelvic floor fitness improves. The tips suggested for each of the following classes are to help you minimize the load upon your pelvic floor if you do choose to participate in them.

PILATES CLASSES

Pilates classes involve low-impact exercises designed to improve your posture, flexibility and muscle strength. These exercises will usually have an appropriate focus upon improving your abdominal muscle control and breathing awareness. Do not be misled into believing that all Pilates exercises will improve your pelvic floor condition. Many Pilates exercises have the potential to place pressure upon your pelvic floor. A number of Pilates exercises develop your outer abdominal muscle strength, which is entirely inappropriate for you if you have or are at risk of pelvic floor dysfunction.

I had been having problems with leakage ever since my last baby. I started going to Pilates classes once a week as I heard that they could help my pelvic floor. My leakage continued to get worse so I started to do the exercises that I could remember at home too. When I saw my physio she suggested that I stop the Pilates for a little while and start pelvic floor exercises. Within a week I was much drier, I couldn't believe the difference.

Cathy, age 41

Inside Out

Pilates tips

♀ Use gently maintained deep abdominal muscle holds and avoid drawing in your abdomen strongly.

♀ Avoid exercises lying on your back and either lifting both your legs or your head and shoulders off the ground, e.g. "The Hundred" and "The Roll Up". Modify double-leg-raise exercises to reduce strain upon your pelvic floor by raising only a single leg at a time and keeping your head down on the mat as shown in Figure 8.1.

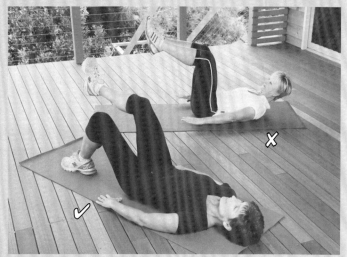

Figure 8.1 Inappropriate double leg raise (right) and modified single leg raise (left)

♀ Avoid exercises supporting your entire body weight through your hands and your feet such as "The Plank". Modify these exercises by supporting your body through your knees rather than your feet, as shown in Figure 7.2.

CIRCUIT TRAINING

Circuit training classes involve various exercise stations, and participants move through these stations at specified time intervals. Circuit classes usually aim to enhance your muscle strength, endurance and aerobic fitness.

Circuit tips
- ♀ Avoid or modify any exercise station with exercises that may compromise your pelvic floor. Many of these are listed under Gym Exercises to Avoid, in Chapter 7.
- ♀ Avoid all abdominal, squat, and leg press machines in equipment-based circuits.
- ♀ Avoid high-impact stations such as running and jumping.

STEP CLASSES

Step classes involve stepping on and off an elevated platform. Participating in step classes will increase your leg strength and may also improve your aerobic fitness and hip bone density.

Step tips
- ♀ Avoid jumping and stepping heavily off your step, especially while holding hand weights.
- ♀ Keep your step height low to reduce the impact on your pelvic floor of stepping down.
- ♀ Do not attempt step classes unless you feel confident in the working ability of your pelvic floor muscles.

WEIGHTED BARBELL CLASSES

Weighted barbell classes incorporate a barbell, free weights/plates and a step platform. Many of the exercises in these classes involve standing and lifting a weighted barbell. These classes are designed to improve your muscle endurance and strength. Remember that the load you lift when you are standing will be transferred to your pelvic floor and it may be difficult for you to modify the exercises in a class situation.

Weighted barbell tips

- ♀ Lift only a manageable weight and never strain when you lift.
- ♀ Avoid exercises such as weighted squats and dead lifts as described in Chapter 7.
- ♀ Avoid abdominal exercises such as weighted sit-ups.
- ♀ Adhere to the "Pelvic Floor Protection Principles" in Chapter 6.
- ♀ Speak with your instructor before the class to advise him or her that there may be exercises you will need to avoid or modify for health reasons.

HIGH-IMPACT EXERCISE CLASSES

High-impact exercise classes involve running and jumping. Avoid these exercises to reduce the impact upon your pelvic floor. High-impact classes are advertised under many different names, e.g. "Fat Buster", "Bodyattack" or "Hi/Lo", so you will need to enquire about the level of high-impact activities in any prospective exercise class. If you are unable to modify the high-impact exercises to low-impact, avoid these classes if you have or are at increased risk of pelvic floor dysfunction.

Key points for exercise classes and your insides

- ♀ Group exercise has many potential health benefits for women.
- ♀ Proceed with caution in exercise classes.
- ♀ Always consider the effect on your pelvic floor of any exercise in any class.
- ♀ Exercise at your own level of comfort and ability.
- ♀ Advise your instructor prior to the class if you need to modify particular exercises.
- ♀ If any exercise exacerbates your symptoms, either modify or cease that exercise altogether.
- ♀ Group exercise classes best suited to protecting your pelvic floor include: water-based, stationary cycle, yoga, exercise ball, dance and Tai Chi classes.
- ♀ Group exercise classes that may contain exercises less suited to protecting your pelvic floor include: Pilates, circuit, step, weighted barbell, and high-impact classes.

9 Home, class or exercise centre?

So now you've made the decision that you want to improve your health and take up some form of exercise. How do you choose between exercising at home, in a group, or perhaps at a fitness centre, and consider your pelvic floor at the same time? There are potential benefits and issues worthwhile considering before you choose to go it alone or sign on the dotted line. The following section is designed to help you match your health needs and personal requirements to the best place for you to exercise. If you choose wisely, you will be more likely to stick with your exercise program and achieve your long-term health goals. The checklist at the end of this chapter will help you to confirm that you have made the right exercise selection for the well-being of your pelvic floor.

PERSONAL CONSIDERATIONS

Considering the following personal factors will help direct you to the appropriate exercise location.

WHAT ARE YOUR HEALTH GOALS?

Identify the specific health gains you want to achieve through exercise. Would you like to:

- ♀ maintain or improve your overall general health?
- ♀ improve your strength and endurance?
- ♀ lose body fat?
- ♀ reduce your stress?
- ♀ prevent or manage a specific illness or disease?
- ♀ improve your flexibility?
- ♀ improve your energy levels?

Make your goals realistic, give yourself a reasonable timeframe in which to achieve them and make them firm by writing them down.

WHAT ARE YOUR HEALTH ISSUES?

Your current and past health issues will also influence your choices. You will need to choose those types of exercise that will promote your health goals and minimize the risk of symptoms and injury to your body.

Do you have problems with your pelvic floor? Do you find that you leak or experience discomfort when you try to exercise? Have you had surgery for a pelvic floor problem? If you *have* had surgery, you should start your exercise program at home under the guidance of your specialist and then gradually progress outside of your home. Make sure that where you choose to exercise allows you to exercise comfortably without compromising your condition or aggravating your symptoms.

HOW GOOD IS YOUR KNOWLEDGE AND UNDERSTANDING?

Do you know what exercise you need to do and how you need to do it to achieve your health goals? If you really understand what you should be doing, you may be someone who will achieve success exercising alone. If you require guidance in meeting your health goals, look around and consider the alternative class and exercise centre options available to you.

HOW STRONG IS YOUR MOTIVATION TO EXERCISE?

How strong is your personal level of motivation to exercise? Are you motivated enough to exercise on your own, or do you prefer to exercise in the company of others? Your own motivation levels will definitely determine how successful you are at sticking with your program and achieving your goals.

WHAT DO YOU ENJOY?

What type of physical activity do you enjoy doing? Choose exercise that you take pleasure in. If you do not like a particular type of exercise, you are unlikely to continue with it long term and it will become a chore. Think back to the types of exercise you have enjoyed in the past. Consider the types of exercise you think you might like to try. You may like to visit different leisure centres or exercise classes to get a feel for what you like doing.

BENEFITS OF HOME, CLASS AND FITNESS CENTRE EXERCISE

BENEFITS OF EXERCISING AT HOME

- Allows you to exercise at your own pace.
- Allows you privacy.
- Gives you the flexibility of exercising when it suits you.
- Time efficient.
- Cost effective.

BENEFITS OF EXERCISE CLASSES

- Usually provide you with quite specific health benefits such as aerobic fitness.
- Provide for guided instruction, potentially reducing your risk of injury and increasing exercise effectiveness.
- Usually cost effective.
- Create an opportunity to meet and mix with others.
- May increase your motivation levels.

BENEFITS OF EXERCISING AT AN EXERCISE CENTRE

- Usually offers a variety of equipment and classes to provide you with a range of health-related benefits.
- The variety of equipment and classes may accommodate a range of health issues.
- Personalized instruction may reduce your risk of injury and increase the effectiveness of your exercises.
- Creates an opportunity to meet and mix with others.
- May increase your motivation levels.
- May provide additional services such as massage and nutritional counselling.

CHOOSING THE RIGHT EXERCISE CLASS OR EXERCISE CENTRE

Let's say you have decided you would prefer to get some instruction and exercise in a group setting rather than at home. There are many general factors that will influence not only where you choose to exercise, but whether you achieve the results you are after and how inclined you are to continue exercising there. These are the types of things worth thinking about for the long-term success of your exercise program.

I had been going to a fitness centre for about 12 months. I was feeling stronger and fitter and generally quite happy with what I was doing there. Some things about the place started to annoy me after a while: the equipment was often broken and it took ages before it was repaired, the air conditioning was never turned on, some of the sweaty people didn't use towels on the equipment and I could never get parking when I was going there after work. I looked around and found another little place close by that is quiet and well maintained.

Sue, age 56

You may wish to consider the following points when visiting a prospective location:

- ♀ What services are offered and do they meet your health needs?
- ♀ What is the atmosphere like?
- ♀ What type of qualifications do the exercise instructors have?
- ♀ Are trained staff willing and available to teach you how to use equipment?
- ♀ Is there provision for an individually prescribed and monitored exercise program?
- ♀ Is there provision for personal training?
- ♀ Does your instructor/trainer have sufficient knowledge and experience in helping you meet your health goals and accommodate your health issues?
- ♀ Is equipment available, clean and well maintained?
- ♀ How convenient is the location for you to get to, and is it close to home and work?

- What is the parking like when you wish to attend?
- Is there air conditioning and when is it turned on?
- What is the price of casual visits and memberships?
- What are the features of membership contracts?
- Is there provision for a trial visit or membership?
- Is the class or centre well established?
- Are there plans to upgrade facilities?

Tips to help you decide

- Visit a number of centres before joining any centre, and compare facilities, services and prices.
- Visit during the hours you anticipate attending that centre.
- Avoid sales pressure as sales of gym memberships can be commission based.
- Speak with someone else you know who attends the centre and ask them about their experiences at the centre.
- If you are considering working with a personal trainer, meet with them first before committing yourself.

Exercise and your pelvic floor checklist

The following checklist has been designed to help you confidently choose the best exercise setting for the well-being of your pelvic floor.

- ☑ I can perform exercise that is low risk for injuring my pelvic floor.
- ☑ I can perform exercise that will cause me minimal symptoms.
- ☑ I can perform low-impact aerobic exercise.
- ☑ I can perform my strength exercises in supported positions.
- ☑ The machine sizes are adjustable and appropriate for my size.
- ☑ The weights are an appropriate size for me to lift.
- ☑ I am comfortable talking to my instructor/trainer.
- ☑ My instructor/trainer will maintain my confidentiality.
- ☑ My instructor/trainer is willing and capable of providing me with safe exercise alternatives.
- ☑ My instructor/trainer is willing to liaise with my health care provider if required.
- ☑ The level of the class is matched to my level of ability.
- ☑ The other class participants have similar ability and experience to mine.
- ☑ The class size allows my instructor to monitor me during class.
- ☑ I feel comfortable around other participants.
- ☑ I can wear clothing I feel comfortable in.
- ☑ The toilets are close by and available if I need them.
- ☑ Change and shower facilities are available if I need them.

Key points for choosing where to exercise

- ♀ Your health goals and health issues will influence the type of exercise your body is best suited to.

- ♀ Ensure that you understand how to achieve your health goals, otherwise seek exercise guidance.

- ♀ Your motivation will influence the success of your program so choose exercise that you enjoy.

- ♀ Home exercise is suited to self-directed and self-paced exercise.

- ♀ Group exercise promotes specific health benefits and guided group instruction.

- ♀ Exercise centres usually provide for a variety of health benefits with equipment, personalized instruction, classes and added services.

- ♀ When deciding where to exercise visit the prospective location.

- ♀ Consider the general factors that may affect whether you achieve the results you are after and continue with your program on a long-term basis.

- ♀ Use your Pelvic Floor Checklist to guide you to choosing the best exercise setting for the well-being of your pelvic floor.

References

[1] Sapsford R, Hodges P, Richardson C, Cooper C, Markwell S (2001) Co-activation of the abdominal and pelvic floor muscles during voluntary exercises. *Neurology and Urodynamics* 20: 31–42.

[2] Hemborg B, Moritz U, Lowing H (1985) Intra-abdominal pressure and trunk muscle activity during lifting. IV: the causal factors of the intra-abdominal pressure rise. *Scandinavian Journal of Rehabilitation Medicine* 17: 25–38.

[3] Thompson J, O'Sullivan P, Briffa N, Neumann P (2006) Differences in muscle activation patterns during voluntary pelvic floor contraction and valsalva manoeuvre. *Neurourology and Urodynamics* 25: 148–155.

[4] Bo K, Aschehoug A (2007) Strength training. In: Bo K, Berghmans B, Morkved S, Van Kampen M (Eds) Evidence-based physical therapy for the pelvic floor. Philadelphia: Butterworth Heinemann Elsevier pp. 119–132.

[5] American College of Sports Medicine and American Heart Foundation (2007) Physical activity and public health: updated recommendation for adults from the American College of Sports Medicine and the American Heart Association. *Medicine & Science in Sports & Exercise* 39: 1423–1434.

[6] American College of Sports Medicine and American Heart Foundation (2007) Physical activity and public health in older adults. Recommendation from the American College of Sports Medicine and the American Heart Association [Special communications: special reports]. *Medicine & Science in Sports & Exercise* 39: 1435–1445.

[7] American College of Sports Medicine (2001) Position stand. Appropriate intervention strategies for weight loss and prevention of weight regain for adults. *Medicine & Science in Sports & Exercise* 33: 2145–2156.

[8] Kenway M (2005) Bone-fit for beginners physiotherapist-designed bone health exercise program (DVD/video), Brisbane: Video Media Productions. www.womensexercise.com.au

[9] American College of Sports Medicine (1998) Position stand. The recommended quantity and quality of exercise for developing and maintaining cardiorespiratory and muscular fitness, and flexibility in healthy adults. *Medicine & Science in Sports & Exercise* 30: 975–991.

[10] Thompson J, O'Sullivan P, Briffa K and Court S (2005) Assessment of pelvic floor movement using transabdominal and transperineal ultrasound. *International Urogynaecology Journal* 16: 285–292.

[11] Neumann P, and Gill V (2002) Pelvic floor and abdominal muscle interaction: EMG activity and intra-abdominal pressure. *International Urogynaecology Journal* 13: 125–132.